A Voice from the Village

A Young Woman's Guide Towards Discovering Her values, sexuality, and self-worth

Carla Jeaneê Bradley

Apostolic Experience Publishing

Apostolic Experience Publishing
8412 Bridlespur Drive
Hazelwood, MO 63942
Phone: 314-479-4888
Web: www.apostolicexperience.com
Email: info@apostolicexperience.com

ISBN 978-0-9790551-3-3

Cover design by Carla Jeaneê Bradley and her son, Miles E. Hill

Illustrations by Carla Jeaneê Bradley

FOR JEANEÊ

MY FIRST "TRUE LOVE"

This book is also dedicated to the Memory of

DENISE PRICE DUDLEY

AND

SUSIE NETTIE BUTLER

Phenomenal Women

Who lived a life of Courage & Service to others

Who were greatly Loved and

Who will be greatly missed

TABLE OF CONTENTS

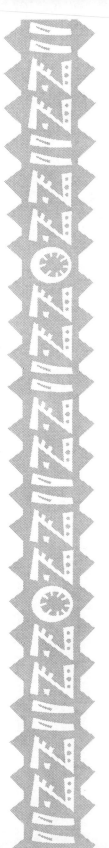

A Note To The Reader....

Ladies:

Many adventures await you as you travel along that mysterious road that leads towards full blown womanhood. And because getting there can be a real trip, I hope this book will provide you with the scenic route. You know, a better view as you travel.

Think of it as a kind of guide book to show you some of the dangerous places that exist along the way and where to find them, in hopes that you never have to go there.

If you get a little lost with some of the words along the way, I hope the glossary in the back of the book will help you get back on track!

My prayer is that in the end, it will also shine a little light on those dark areas so you can see them more clearly, and avoid those detours that can lead to a dead end street.

At best, I hope to persuade at least one young lady to honor and value herself, make wiser choices because of it, and live the glorious life she was meant to live. Then my work here is done. I hope that young lady will be you!

Have a wonderful, remarkable journey!

Carla

CHAPTER ONE

The Purpose of "A Voice" and the Village Connection

There are a few things that I hope you can take away with you from this book. Mainly, that you alone have control over your bodies and your mind. If you don't take control over them, someone else will. My prayer is that in the end, you might have a broader perspective with regards to your sexuality, and that most importantly, you will have faith that you and God are enough. YOU ARE ENOUGH!!!

There is so much that goes along with being sexually active. Shame, guilt, worry, pain, rejection, humiliation, self-loathing, emptiness, just to name a few. And the degradation! (deg-ra-day-shun: "the act of de-valuing or of putting someone down, giving them a "beat-down" physically, emotionally and spiritually, and then spitting on them. Then adding one last kick while they're down, just cuz you can.) We must be ready (meaning mature enough) to handle all of the emotions that come along for the ride. I just thought at your age, you are going through enough already, so I'm just trying to help a sister out.

It is important to note that the feelings you may be experiencing are natural and happen to almost everyone. They are not just happening to you, although sometimes it feels that way. Although you may feel strange and all alone at times, you are far from being either. It's all part of the changes our bodies go through as women on the road to womanhood.

And you are never alone.

Those feelings... the ones you have that you really can't explain... if not acted upon, will not kill you, no matter how much you think they will.

On the contrary, acting upon them could very well kill you. Literally or spiritually. If you don't have a spirit that radiates love, illuminates confidence, and soars towards pure joy, then a part of you is dead already.

With AIDS, HIV, and other sexually transmitted diseases (STD's) on the rise, mostly due to unprotected sexual contact, and mostly in your age bracket, you really need to ask yourself, "is being with this guy really worth dying for?" You know, end of story, game over, you lose, people wearing black and crying, 'cause "you won't be coming back no more, no more, no more, no more?" Is he worth *that* kind of dying for? Is he worth your life?

Aren't You?

Is satisfying your curiosity worth leaving your family, friends, and life behind no matter how much they get on your nerves? Is a few minutes (Yes, that's all it takes) of *maybe* a good time worth your whole entire life?

These are the questions you need to ask yourself when you start getting all hot and bothered and stuff. And the answer is "No!" He is not worth all that. NO ONE IS! No matter how F-I-N-E you think he is. No matter how he makes you feel.

The purpose of this book is to help you to see that you have value. You are worth so much more than you could even begin to imagine! All you need to do is just believe that you are. It's really just that simple.

The Village Connection

It has been said that it takes a village to raise a child. That means that a child who comes into this world is not the sole responsibility of the parents who brought that child forth, but also the responsibility of all others around who may have an impact on that child's life. It is the extended family to the extreme, looking out for and providing guidance to every child in any way that could be helpful and beneficial.

Unfortunately, in today's society, that "village" has virtually been destroyed. A lot of neighborhoods don't have strong communities anymore: we barely know our neighbors. We don't look out for each other the way we should, and people are barely accountable for themselves, let alone someone else's child.

The days of being spanked by a neighbor and then later "beat down" by your parents are gone for good; and although you may be happy about that, the truth is, there are not a lot of people looking out for you. Few people are leading you and guiding you in positive directions and away from future problems. The help is out there, but it's usually not next door anymore.

Even our extended families are in trouble, and so you, as young women, are left without a lot of people around that have your back. There is not a society of women stepping up and giving you the 411 on things that may be helpful for you to know, or that could save you from years of heartache or major therapy.

So that's what this book is: A Voice from the world village. I know there is a whole community of Sister Villagers out there who also want to help you because when I told them about this book that you are now holding in your hands, they'd say, "Girl...make sure you tell them this." Or "Ohhh, do you talk about that?" Or simply, "Carla, please make sure you include such and such, because that really would have helped me make different choices in my life."

I feel an obligation as a member of the Village to do something about the situation that my young sisters are facing. Some of your spirits are so wounded they could audition for a remake of the *Thriller* video. I had to do whatever I could to help elevate your spirit. That is how this book was born. I hope that you will consider it as my gift to you, from women everywhere, to help you make better choices in your life.

As one voice from the village that still exists in the hearts and minds of many, all that I'm trying to get you to see, is that a few minutes, and a bad decision, can totally change the course of your life. Or even end it. I hope to give you some tools necessary to make better decisions, wiser choices, or at least put some things on your beautiful mind.

That's why I'm putting the information out there, offering some suggestions, and hopefully answering some questions along the way. I hope that you will have more knowledge and information about the choices that are available, and the consequences of each.

Knowledge is Power. How you use that knowledge is Wisdom. Do whatever you can to gain more of each. And don't worry... 'cause I got your back.

CHAPTER TWO

Our Value – Then & Now

Back in the Day

Hundreds and hundreds of years ago, from the beginning of time, really, wars have been fought, empires were gained or destroyed, and men would risk everything, even kingdoms, over a woman. The desire to possess her and be the first to penetrate her virtue (get some) drove men into battle or death.

Marriages were arranged, and young girls were promised, even as babies, to men from "good" families as future husbands. A woman was considered so valuable in fact, that she was often traded for or purchased with gold, land, cattle, or anything that was considered valuable at that time. Nowadays, these knuckleheads don't even call you back!

We can't talk about the beginning unless we talk about the very beginning, and the woman who pretty much screwed it up for all of us. That woman of course, was the very first woman, Eve. She just had to listen to that old snake (and we all know a few of them) and then she talked Adam into going along with her, even though he too, knew eating from that Forbidden Tree was wrong.

Her power of persuasion, by whatever method she used, and bringing another down with her even though she knew better, is the reason that women today birthe babies in a painful way instead of a joyous one, as explained in Genesis 3:16. Had it not been for her giving in to temptation, we probably wouldn't get cramps either. Darn her.

Her act created the "curse" of which women speak, because she made it painful to be a woman. We are still paying for her first mistake. We know we can tempt and seduce men, and use our feminine ways to sometimes get them to do things we both know is wrong. We have since the very beginning. We also know that most men wouldn't deny a woman if they offered themselves to them. So why do we continue to try to tempt them?

Sometimes our mind shifts from focusing on and being thankful for what we do have to stressing out over the one thing that we don't have. The desire to have what we want takes over us completely, and we can hardly think of anything else. Our minds can get so completely consumed with that one thing we want, we don't have room in our heads for anything else, including sanity.

Think back to a time when there was something that you wanted. I mean really, really wanted. You wanted it so bad—you just knew for sure that you would fall out and die if you didn't get it. And then what? Either one of two things happened.

A. You didn't get what you wanted and you are still here and breathing, or

B. You did get it and you found out that it really wasn't worth the emotional roller coaster ride it took you on in the first place.

And where is it now? See what I'm saying?

If it's a guy that you feel this way about, give it some time. Don't give in to those "I want him and just got to have him" feelings, and pretty soon, you will see that you were just temporarily blinded by this obsession to have what you didn't have already. Three words you must remember when you feel this way: It will pass.

After a while, (like the next week or so) you'll probably look at him and scratch your head in amazement and wonder what made you think you had to have him in the first place. Trust me.

Practice a little patience, observe him closely, but not through dreamy eyes. Watch him through eyes that are wide open to the truth, and you'll soon find out that he, just like those other things you just had to have, really isn't worth the hype. (Or hyperventilation that your body goes through trying to catch your breath and slow down your heart beat every time you see him. That will pass too.)

The major difference between the guy and the "thing" you wanted is that once you finally do get the "thing," heartbreak doesn't usually follow. A little letdown maybe, but getting the guy and then finding out the truth, which is one of the following, can be a very painful experience:

A. That he only wanted you for sex

B. That he's with you because of a bet he'd made

C. He really doesn't even like you back

D. He is a complete and total idiot

E. All of the above

That "I've just got to have it no matter what" feeling that Eve experienced is typical of all of us. Our desires, like hers, can be so strong at times that we don't even think of the consequences that could come about for getting what we desire and long for. We can give up so much, in an instant, just to have that one thing that we don't have. We continue to this very day to show we are her descendents by consistently repeating her same mistake.

That's some powerful stuff if you really think about it. One woman, the very first woman in fact, is still affecting millions of women. Women are some powerful beings! What you need to know (that Eve failed to realize) is that desires can be controlled. Patience is the key. And most importantly, your actions will also affect the lives of many others as well and not always in a good way. We need to be strong where she was not. Especially now that we know what can happen!

Imagine how life could have been for women had she just refused temptation... No cramps, no labor pains in childbirth. We may not even have had to have periods every month! Who knows? Imagine how life could be for future generations if you begin to resist those desires and longings and choose to do the right thing instead of the wrong one.

How Times Have Changed

As we move closer to the present, but still back in the day, you should know that in Africa, prior to slavery, and in other countries and cultures around the world, promiscuity was not allowed. Sometimes girls were married in their very early teens, (or younger) but either way, you were a virgin when you married. Period. If you were not, you brought great shame to your family, the family name, and maybe your entire village.

Preparation for the wedding ceremony was a preparation for womanhood. The Elder women would gather with you and teach you all of the things you should know about your duties, your roles, and how to be a wife to your husband. There was none of that "Just figure it out as you go along" stuff. Other women around you instructed you, so you kinda knew what to expect.

Some societies in Nigeria, (like the Hausa and Nupe tribes) also did not allow sexual contact of any kind before marriage. There would be no spoiling of the ceremonies that marked a turning point in a young woman's life.

Any man who took a woman's virginity and they were not married, was treated as a common thief. He had stolen her future. He brought shame to himself and his family, and in some cases was even treated like a criminal.

Now think about slavery. Imagine what it was like to be the property of someone else, and to be used for the satisfaction of the slave owner, his family members, his boys, or whoever else he had in mind, whenever the mood hit him. It didn't matter how old you were, whether you loved someone or not, were married or not, or whether you even wanted to or not. Not doing it was not an option.

It didn't matter if the guy was some big fat, foul smelling, bald-headed-but-hairy-everywhere-else-man with only two teeth in his head and both of them were rotten. It didn't matter who he was, how he was, what he looked like, or how you felt. You had no choice in the matter. No say at all.

As property, we could be used as many things, including sexual favors. There was absolutely nothing that we could do about it. Even the men in our lives were powerless to step in and stop it from happening. It was just the way it was. We were voiceless. Powerless. We had to keep our feelings about it silent or face severe beatings or even death if we resisted or refused.

Because of this, Black women especially were believed to be always sexually available, even though we were not always willing participants.

Our value as women continued to decline through time. Look at the way women are portrayed today in music videos for example. Those images only perpetuate (meaning, make it never end) the myth that we are highly sexual beings. We not only "shake what our Mommas gave us" we even shake the things we got on our own (breast implants, hair weaves and other fake stuff that makes us look like God never intended us to look like). Our booty cheeks are all but totally exposed, and breasts and nipples are everywhere, except inside a shirt.

We throw our half-dressed bodies and body parts all over men, licking suggestively on our finger as if we could win a contest for our abilities, and trying to tease them into pretending that it was a part of him we would like to do that to instead. And we don't even know him!

First of all, let's not kid ourselves, ladies. There are some talents that we should be proud of, but they are usually ones we can put on a job application, and that is not one of them. Secondly, why would you want a guy to be attracted to you for that... being a penis cleaner I mean? But most importantly, what is the overall message you are sending (loud and very clear) to these guys?

For a ride in a fancy car, some "bling-bling" around your neck, or just a chance to be with a guy for what he can (but not necessarily will) give you in exchange for your body, you would sell yourself and other women that cheap??? Sometimes they do all this for some scary looking guy that they normally wouldn't even look at twice. And they certainly wouldn't want to run into him in a dark alley. And they certainly wouldn't bring him home to meet their parents.

They parade around these guys with this "come and get it" look on their face, showing all of their goods (and even some not-so-goods), and slither up and down a Brother's body, enticing him in sexual ways. The message that they (the women in these videos) are sending is basically this, "Baby, you can have me for a song... or a chance to be seen in a video. I am not worth more than how I look, so who cares what you do to me, or what comes after you use me."

The music industry has stooped to an all-time low in order to further devalue and degrade women. I hope you can open your minds long enough and wide enough to look beyond the latest heart-throb singing or rapping, or even the funky beat. Look beyond the images of over-exposure of our body parts, and hopefully you will see that our sisters are being exploited. And you, girlfriend, are part of her family. Those women don't make any money dancing in those videos. A lot of them have to do some of the same things you see them pretending to do, (only not with a finger), just to be on the video in the first place! You better ask somebody!

How they are viewed and treated affects how all women are viewed and treated. We are so much more than sexual objects and our bodies are beautiful, yes. That's why we should not be shared with every Tom, Dick, or Harry just for their pleasure. Neither should we allow those men and others to think about us in freaky ways either.

Thoughts are very powerful things. Sometimes a sexual thought about you from another based on some teasing, tempting, or suggestion, either real or imagined, can lead to an obsession to make that thought a reality. And trust me, you may not be ready to go where his mind has been. You were just flattered that someone was thinking of you in that way. Don't be flattered, sweetie. Be afraid.

Some of his thoughts could be dangerous for you if they are in the wrong man's head. Don't give them anything to work with. They pick up signals from us that we don't even know we're sending.

Don't be flirty, expose yourself, or engage in sexual conversations, especially with someone you've just met, or someone you may be chatting with online. They already have in their mind images of us from the women they've seen in music videos and in other areas of Porn (Pornography) and some see us exactly that way already: easy, ready, and always available. You should not want to be seen or even thought of in this way.

Understanding Our Value

So what does all that past stuff have to do with me today, you ask? Hopefully, it's to get you to see the value in what you are. If you don't give value to yourself, someone else will put a value on you.

THE MORE VALUABLE YOU ARE THE LESS LIKELY YOU ARE TO BE USED.

That statement really has two different meanings. One way to interpret it is that your value decreases the more you have been *used*. The more you allow men to use you-for sex, for money, or for baby making, the less valuable you appear to be.

Think of a pricey collector's item such as a Special Limited Edition hand-painted porcelain doll. You would be shocked, I'm sure, if you knew how much of a collector's item those dolls are, and how much they are worth!

The actual value of the doll is dramatically decreased if the seal on the box is broken and she was actually taken out of the box. If she had been played with, (and you know how we like to play in the hair, take the clothes off and stuff like that) she could no longer get top price.

In fact, the doll is probably no longer even considered a Collectors Item. She would be just another doll. She would only be worth what was paid for her at the time of purchase, or even less than that.

Once the seal is broken and she has been handled, her value immediately decreased. Even if she was only played with for a minute and you couldn't even tell, and was put back exactly as she was found, it wouldn't even matter.

Not that you are for sale or anything, or that you should just be kept on display admired and collected, so, please don't get me wrong for what I'm about to say. I'm just saying, you should think of your self in much the same way. If your value goes down when you are removed from your box (of innocence and purity) - and your seal is broken (you lose your virginity), then all I'm saying is: Don't let anyone play with you unless they plan on keeping you!

Besides, you can never repair the seal once broken, and you will never be exactly the way you were before, even if you think people can't tell you've been played with. Men won't just try to play in your hair, and for sure they won't be taking off your clothes for the same reason we would. The box of course would be ripped into several pieces, and the seal? Forget about it! They sure will.

Try to think of yourself as a Collector's Item, just waiting for the right guy to come along and appreciate you for the treasure that you are, and the value of which you have. Someone who would lovingly and carefully open the box and won't mess you up to the point where no one else wants to play with you.

The other way of looking at that statement (The More Valuable you are the Less you are used) can be more empowering. But it takes a little work to get there. Think of it this way:

IF YOU PLACE A HIGH VALUE ON YOURSELF, AND KNOW HOW VALUABLE YOU ARE, YOU ARE NOT AS LIKELY TO ALLOW YOURSELF TO BE USED.

You are always worth a lot more than you think. You are priceless! What you are and what you have is far too valuable to be given away for nothing. Literally, nothing!

Girlfriend, as a woman, you are worth so much more than you could ever imagine! At the very least you are worth a man's commitment to you in marriage. You know? A promise to be a part of his future and not just his past.

You are worthy to be loved, cherished, and adored. Right now, many of you have no idea what that feels like. Some of you may think you do, but just believe me when I tell you that at this point in time, unless those feelings are coming to you from a loving father, (or father-figure) you have no idea what it's like.

Little girls who grow up feeling the love and security from a father, as well as discipline and concern, tend to look for mates that closely resemble what they've experienced. From that relationship, they know how a man should treat them and usually, don't settle for anything less.

If you are among the very select few who have a man like this in your life, love him, appreciate him and respect him because he is setting the standard for what you should be looking for in a future mate. I know for a fact that there are men like this with their little girls because I have actually met a few of them. So I know they exist.

Honor him by showing him that you get it. That you will not settle for any less than the love and adoration that he has shown to you. And give him a hug for me and tell him I said "Hats off for holding it down and representing like a dad is supposed to represent." You are blessed to have him in your life. Don't ever forget that or take it for granted.

If, on the other hand, you are like myself and so many other countless women who did not have a man like that in our lives, we pay a high price for that. We are always looking for love (in all the wrong places) or someone to fill that void—that empty space we feel by not having a father's love and tenderness in our lives.

There seems to be this huge, gigantic hole in us and trying to fill it becomes our unconscious desire. We know there is something missing and we tend to fall for any man who gives us a little attention, makes us feel special or tells us that he loves us. Whether he means any of it or not.

What we are missing is the love, security, protection, and comfort of a man who truly loves and cares for us. We are searching for that missing piece in our lives where we are valued as little girls and young women. (Being spoiled a little bit wouldn't hurt either).

A man's penis alone will not fill up that empty space. In fact, that's not even where the hole is! A man's body part can not fill the void you feel by not having a father in your life, although many will try.

Honor yourself, love yourself, respect yourself and give value to yourself. In time, God will make you whole. Don't ask for respect. Demand it. Someone worthy of you and all you have to offer will come along. And hopefully, you'll be ready and able to recognize it when it does.

This question came to my mind, and I couldn't get it out of my head. What made women and womanhood more valuable in the past—worthy of lost empires, declaration of wars, treasures gained and lost, and countless losses of life—than how we are valued today?

The answer was really quite simple. It lies in how we as women treat ourselves and how we treat our bodies. And, in how society treats women (and our bodies). Getting to the mystery that is between our legs is no longer a sought-after victorious and sweet honor to possess because we've made it that way. It is far too available.

You can get some over here, or get some over there. You can even see some on TV anytime, all the time, even prime time. Anything that's free and easy and available for everybody somehow isn't so special anymore. Free is good at first, but after a while it's usually not worth keeping. Especially if everyone else has the same thing!

Women aren't valued as much because we don't even value our own selves! We don't even take the time to get to know who we are and what we are about, or supposed to be about. We are never satisfied with ourselves, and are always trying to make changes. You know what I mean, in our hair, our bodies, our ways. We've got too much of "this" and not enough of "that." We hate ourselves, but want everyone else to love us.

How we are valued is a direct reflection of what we do to our own selves. When we start really loving ourselves, treating ourselves with respect, focusing on our positive qualities instead of our negative ones, others will fall in line. Or they'll just need to step out of it! But first, we need to show them where that line should start. Respect yourself, and they will too.

We can't even get mad for real when we end up being treated the way we treat ourselves—like trash bins just waiting for someone to come and dump all of their stuff. You know, like their egos, attitudes and lustful ideas. And we just take it all in as if it's okay. But when we allow men to dump into us, their semen contains the stuff that contains the makings of a baby, and could possibly contain disease as well.

Unless you consider yourself to be a trash can, don't allow any trash to be put inside of you. That's not what the hole was made for anyway! Make *pride* be your landfill to fill that space and stop the dumping!!! What makes them think we want what they don't even want their own self! You know what I mean?

But that is exactly what we are inviting guys to do when we chase after them. "Come on over here and dump on me, dump in me, fill me with your waste", we beg. So a word to the wise… Don't chase him, don't pursue him, and don't throw your stuff at him, suggestively or otherwise. He may act like he likes it now, but then he'll wonder how many other guys you've done the same thing to. And soon it will all come back and smack you in the face. And you will become what you're full of. Save all of that for marriage, and then what is deposited in you will not be trash, but a blessing from God.

Let the man do what a man is supposed to do. We don't need to advertise… or give away free samples. Everybody already knows what we have, and everybody knows it's good. Let the man chase after you. You would think so much better of yourself if he made the first move anyway. Don't doubt your worthiness by making a move on him.

In the book of Proverbs, Chapter 31, it says that a woman (wife) of noble character is worth far more than rubies. If you purpose your life to be about good character, truth, and helping not harming others, then know that your value will be worth far more than a collection of rare and precious gems. And that is exactly what you are!

THE VALUE OF WOMEN AROUND THE WORLD

Just to give you an idea of how different life is for women elsewhere, outside of the USA, and show the value of women around the world, in the present day, I thought I'd share some facts about things you may, or may not have been aware of. Hopefully, it will make you appreciate being a woman born in the United States. More importantly, I hope it will make you value the choices you are *allowed* to make by having the rights that we have.

♥ Women and little girls to this day, continue to be gang-raped, taken from their homes and villages, and forced into sexual slavery by rebel groups along the Congo River. It is a practice that has been going on for years.

♥ Due to the overcrowding in China, the Government has implemented population control, allowing each married couple only one child. As a result, Chinese baby girls [not as desirable as a male heir in many cases] are left abandoned on the streets, or basically thrown away. Orphanages are filled to capacity. Some are literally dying from neglect.

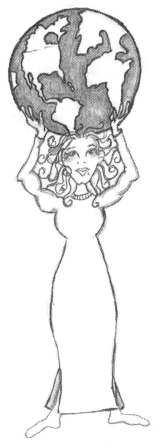

♥ Female circumcision, the removal of parts of the vagina that would make sex pleasurable for women, is still being practiced in certain African cultures, even if the women reside in the United States. Not only is sex displeasing, it is also painful and the women are more prone to infections.

♥ Little girls in Taiwan, Brazil, and other impoverished areas all over the world are forced into prostitution, or sold, sometimes by their very own parents into the black market to be used for whatever, by whomever, in exchange for income.

23

This is just a small example of the way women [our sisters] are being treated around the world today. Women are clearly not valued as much as they use to be, or even should be, especially in other parts of the world. You should be aware of these girls and young women and the lives they are forced to live, because they unfortunately, don't have a choice. But you do.

We can change all that. If enough of us take a stand to demand better treatment, or stop buying products that degrade women, then eventually, there will be a shift—a complete change of direction and the music industries and others that exploit women will have to sit up and take notice. We can even force our government to acknowledge the brutality of women in other parts of the world, and try to put a stop to it.

We can stand up for ourselves as young women and recognize the beauty of the power in numbers. We can demand to be treated with the respect we deserve, and also demand a more accurate portrayal of how we really are.

As Emancipated Slave and Civil Rights Activist Sojourner Truth said, while speaking at the Women's Rights Convention in 1851:

> *"If the first woman God ever made was strong enough to turn the world upside down all alone, these women together ought to be able to turn it back, and get it right side up again."*

We have the power to determine how men treat us. All we need is the desire for change. Let's do it for Ms. Truth. Let's turn this thing back around to a time when women were valued and worth something! She did not speak up for the rights of women and risk her life time and time again just so we could dance half naked in a music video.

She and many others fought for our freedom so that we would no longer be treated as voiceless property. She wanted us, as women, to have the right to be treated as a human being, with freedom to make choices about our bodies, our families and our lives. She is one of many great women who have proved that one person really can make a difference. Her spirit, strong, committed, and revolutionary, still resides in us all.

How Much Are You Worth?

Try to give some serious thought to these questions. It works best if you write down your answers and not just think of them in your head. Look back at your answers again after finishing the book, and see if your value has gone up or if there are any changes you would make to your original thoughts.

1. If you could put any price on your head, what would it be? How much would you cost if you were for sale?

2. Why? (And "Because" is not an answer.)

3. What if someone offered you money for your life? How much would that be worth?

4. Why is your life worth that?

5. What if the price you were offered meant that you would belong to someone else, and be a sex slave or a breeder and will spend the rest of your days being used, mistreated and looked down upon by the rest of society? How much would you cost then?

6. How much money would it take to persuade you to allow someone to give you a disease to which there is no cure, just to conduct an experiment to see the pain and agony your body goes through and the length of time it takes before you die? How much would you cost to be used for scientific purposes?

CHAPTER THREE

The Most Precious Gift

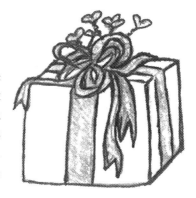

In the last chapter we explored some of the value in our virtue and the great lengths men would go to get it. Men continue to think that they have what is desired, that it is their penis that we want. That we crave. When in fact, the flip-side is actually the truth. It has always been.

We need to get over on the other side... and start seeing the vagina the way it deserves to be seen. As the powerful, desirable, and sacred force that it really is. And we have the power to change that.

Have you ever heard the joke about the two little girls, sitting on the front stoop, talking to each other about the things they wanted in life?

The first little girl says, "When I grow up, I want to have a brand new shiny car, a closet full of clothes and shoes, and a purse full of money." The other girl thinks for a minute, and says with absolute confidence, "All I want when I grow up is a patch of hair right here," she says, pointing to the area where her thighs meet.

Puzzled, the other girl said "A patch of hair? Why would you want that?" The other girl put one hand on her hip and in a matter of fact way said "Well, my sister has all of those things you said you wanted, and she said with this, (pointing again) she can have whatever she wants!"

Yes, your vagina can be that powerful. It can be so good it can get you all those things and more. Like death, disease, or an unplanned new member of society.

The story about the two little girls makes a good point. Everyday, you sit on something so powerful, it's almost magic. And it certainly has magical powers. Sometimes it can act like a magnet and seem to draw a lot of men to it. Sometimes it can make a man do crazy things (but not always in a good way). A lot of men will want it, but not if everyone else has already had it. The desire to have you will greatly increase if they know that they are going where no one else has been, where they can be the first to explore. Don't let anyone ever take advantage of that.

But it is even more powerful than that. The vagina is the key to the entrance of your heart. What goes on in there is directly connected to our emotions, our hearts.

For men, the act itself is not unlike how they are in general. Everything is on the outside. With men, young and old, their emotions are not tied to their penises; everything with them is surface stuff. This is not unlike the penis itself, which hangs on the outside of his body.

For women, sex with us is internal. It happens on the inside of us. We allow the man to actually insert his external body part into our bodies, and for a time, he becomes a part of us. Part of who he is is inside of who we are. He literally pierces through and penetrates our weakened outer barrier and invades our very being. And it forever changes who we are.

Long after the act itself is over, and thoughts of him are a distant memory, he can never be forgotten because he will always be a part of us. And a part of our history. Whether he rocked our world or not.

We just opened up, and let someone become an actual part of us. He's in there, 'hanging out' with our insides. He could never be any closer to us than that.

We allow him to enter into a sacred place that opens up to the area where life is created, maintained, and brought forth.

LIFE

God works his magic, and women sustain it and bring his plan into physical reality through our womb. And out of our vagina. A gift through our Gift. You cannot allow just anybody to poke around in there! That place is sacred!

While it's true that without man and his sperm a baby cannot be made, without woman, there would be no place to carry it. And where does that child grow? Exactly. You get the picture.

It is all internal for us, and therefore, the emotions and feelings we have in our heart are directly connected to that experience, and should therefore only be entered into within the realm of marriage.

God made women to bring life to the world. He gave us a gift that through us brings forth the gift of life. That is the original purpose of "getting busy" (having intercourse) in the first place.

But just because we can make a baby, it doesn't mean that we have to. Especially when we're not ready and the guy is not worthy. Our gift does not have to be the gift that keeps on giving!

We can never penetrate a man and become a part of him like he becomes a part of us. The hole in his penis is much too small for that. But seriously, it just wasn't made to be that way. We cannot expect him to feel for us the way we feel for him. We may be just another warm place to stick his stuff for a minute. Sometimes, we are a much too convenient place.

Every time you engage in a sexual act, you are actually giving away a piece of yourself, and there are only so many pieces to a whole. You are a woman, not a puzzle. Shouldn't the person you are giving the precious gift of yourself to at least be worthy enough to receive it?

Think about what he will do with the gift he receives from you, that piece of you they take. Will he throw it away, discard it like trash? Will he compare it to his other pieces and add it to his collection? Will he share it with his friends and invite them to come get a piece too? Or, will he cherish it for the precious gift and beautiful treasure that it is?

If you give away too much of yourself, there won't be much of you left. You will be just a shell of the woman you were created to be with parts of you missing that will never be returned.

A whole of something is better than a piece of anything (except for trouble of course). If you're not careful about who you share your treasure with, a whole lot of trouble is what you may end up with.

He should want all of you—not just a piece! You have so much more to offer than what's between your legs. If you recognize that, he will too.

You need all of your pieces in order to be a whole person

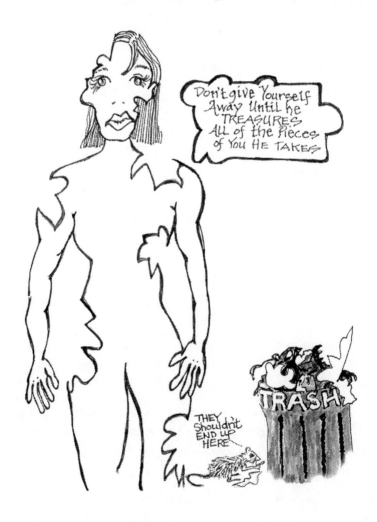

That's why you need to know that the man you carefully choose to allow in isn't just looking for another warm spot. You should know that he wants the total package of who you are and what you're about. That he cares about you, your feelings, your joys and your pains. That he is 'in' to you in more ways than one.

Women have been using their bodies to get money or other material things since Biblical times. I am not suggesting that you use your precious body to acquire things, I am simply pointing out the power that it has to do so. They don't call prostitution the world's oldest profession for nothing.

Now, some of your sisters are selling themselves way too cheap or even just giving themselves away. It could even be you.

You should in fact, be trying to get all of those things the little girls in the joke were talking about on your own, with your own money. Men like that. And it should be money that you have earned by using your brain and not your body. You'll like that.

If you want to really be attractive to a man, have your stuff together, and show him you can take care of yourself. I'm mostly talking to the older girls right now, who may be working part-time or during breaks from school.

I'm not saying to take care of him, though. You know, like always treating him or him and his boys when you hang out. Or always being the one to buy him gifts and things. Men are supposed to take care of themselves. Besides, we don't need to buy anyone or pay anyone to be with us. We just have it like that!!

If you are in a situation like that, or know someone who is, get out of it because you are just being used. And misused. That is not how it is supposed to be!

What I'm talking about is being in a position of not feeling obligated to a man for anything, at anytime, or feeling like you owe him something in exchange for something he did or gave to you. Even if that means having enough money to call a cab if you need to in order to get out of an uncomfortable situation. If you don't need him for anything, you will find that it not only gives you a sense of power, but that it can also make you more attractive.

If you use wisdom and make responsible choices, you can easily have what your heart desires. Yes, having a vagina can get you all sorts of things. Including a baby or a casket. The choice is yours, so choose responsibly.

To truly honor this precious gift, you should strive to keep it free of disease, free of strangers who don't belong, and sealed until marriage. In other words, Keep it Clean, Keep it Sacred, and Keep it Tight!

CHAPTER FOUR

Protect Your Rep... (utation)

Have you ever heard the expression "Your reputation precedes you"? This means that people know of you, and quite often, form opinions of you, well before they ever lay eyes on you.

People knew of Jesus and the miracles he'd performed before they saw him or touched the hem of his garment. People knew him because of what they'd heard because people spread the word about him. His reputation, the kind of man he was and what he stood for, was introduced to them long before they saw him.

In the present day, when asked to think of a powerful, inspirational woman whose purpose is to make the world a better place than when she found it, most of you may think of Oprah. Her reputation of humanitarian efforts and all that she strives to do for people here and in other countries precedes her.

What is the reputation that precedes you? What could people be saying about you that introduces you to others that do not know you? Now we both know that girls will be girls, and they're gonna talk. And so can boys—they can make some stuff up and spread lies just like the next girl. The best way to avoid this is to stay clear of any situations that would even give the appearance that a rumor about you may be true. Even the Bible warns us to "Stay away from all appearances of evil." But your real reputation is behind all the lies and petty rumors.

For example, let's just say that some guy started spreading a rumor that they had been with you, or you had done this or that. If his friends or anyone else can say, "Her? Man that girl won't even talk about sex, or even let me kiss her." Because you had stayed away from appearances of evil or even "flirty" behavior, the guy trying to spread the rumor would not have a leg to stand on.

Others would doubt him simply because what he says does not match the reputation that went before you.

If, on the other hand, you have been known to talk a lot about sex, or have been seen hanging out with various guys, even kissing one or two of them, the rumors about you may appear to be true, even if they are not.

Although I love men dearly, a large number of them tend to exaggerate and stretch the truth a bit. They learn this very early on, and unfortunately, the stories get bigger as they do.

You have heard, I'm sure, about men and their "fish tales". You know, "I caught a fish that was this big" they say as they stretch their arms out as far as they can go. Needless to say, the fish somehow got away, and there is no photo to prove whether it's true or not.

By the same token, if you were interested in some guy, and let's say you kissed him, and nothing else. To his friends, a lot more would have happened. For them, it's like a sport. It's like scoring: he who gets the most points wins.

What you have is far more valuable, and hopefully, you will eventually find someone who isn't into playing games or keeping score. When you are valued for who you are and not how far you'll go, you are the ultimate winner.

Since a guy may say things have happened between the two of you that didn't really happen, he may then try to force you into a situation so he can be right about it. His reputation is now on the line. This could be dangerous for you if he tries to take you by force, and very painful for you if you continue to reject him and then he leaves you. There are four words you can say if he leaves you for not putting out: Oh Well. See Ya!

Always remember, your reputation is at stake, (not to mention far more important than his) and you always have the right to stop unwanted advances. And if he's willing to leave you if he can't get any, then what does that say about his motives to be with you in the first place? Exactly. Better to find out now rather than later, and believe me, it's a lot less painful.

Hopefully, you will see sooner rather than later, that you made the right choice by honoring yourself, and standing your ground. After all, isn't your reputation more valuable?

Protect your Rep by maintaining a respectable self-image and a firm commitment to abstinence. It can be kind of hard not even thinking about it at first until you really commit yourself. Don't beat yourself up. We are, after all, only human. And we are made of flesh, and flesh can get weak. It gets easier with time (and a little prayer for strength wouldn't hurt).

The only thing worse than being a virgin and having a reputation as a "ho", is then giving in to it by becoming what you are accused of. Whether anybody knows the truth or not, you do, and that's enough. Hold firm to your commitment, don't become what you're accused of, and eventually, the truth will come out.

Have the reputation that you don't just put out for anybody and that you're waiting for marriage. Then the guys may say something like "She must think she's special or something." Then you can smile because now they know something that you already knew.

They will also know that the guy who does finally get the honor will have to be something special too. They will try really hard to be that special one, so be forewarned. Like I said, the best way to get the attention of a guy is to not give him any of yours. (Attention I mean).

Protect your reputation at all costs, because unlike a bad hair day, it can be something that stays with you forever. It can become a permanent label advertising who you are, whether it's true or not. And it can greatly effect the way you see yourself, treat yourself, or allow others to treat you.

Most importantly, don't become what you are labeled (unless of course it's a good thing) because you feel unable to remove it. Those negative labels even our own families can put on us when they refer to us, by using terms like "the fat one", "the greedy one", or "the one that ain't got no sense."

Don't accept these labels people put on you no matter who they are! If you accept them they will begin to stick and pretty soon you might find yourself believing them as well.

When people try to assign a label to you, look around as if you are trying to see who they are talking about. Or say to them, "that is not me and I wish you would stop calling me that."

If you can't repel them and stop them from coming, you can peel them off and make new ones for yourself. "The smart one." The successful one." "The one who is going to do great things."

Once you get those in your spirit and start believing them, others will see in you what you believe yourself to be. And a new Rep can emerge.

People are always talking or being talked about and labeled. Unfortunately, that's just human nature. Make sure when they talk about you it's with pride and admiration rather than something bad or negative.

Make sure the rep that precedes you is one that truly represents and reflects who you are and what you stand for. When you begin to believe it, others will too.

ZIZIZIZIZIZIZIZIZIZIZIZIZIZIZIZIZIZIZIZIZIZIZIZIZIZIZIZIZIZIZIZIZIZIZ

Exercise

Think of some of the labels that others have tried to assign to you. Write down as many as you can remember on index cards or pieces of paper. Think about how each one made you feel, and who was trying to assign them to you.

For each of the negative labels that attempted to attach themselves to you, replace each one with either the complete opposite, or something else that better suits your spirit. Write those down as well in the same manner.

Rip those negative labels up into as many tiny pieces as you can. Stomp on them, spit on them, flush them down the toilet, or whatever you can do to physically destroy and eliminate them and the feelings that went along with those labels.

Begin to be the new label that you have assigned. Every time someone tries to put a negative label on you, in your mind replace it with the new one you have selected, and forgive that person for their ignorance. (Be careful though... you don't want to assign labels either).

Watch the change in your attitude, behavior and level of self-confidence as it improves and begins to reflect your new image.

ZIZIZIZIZIZIZIZIZIZIZIZIZIZIZIZIZIZIZIZIZIZIZIZIZIZIZIZIZIZIZIZIZIZIZ

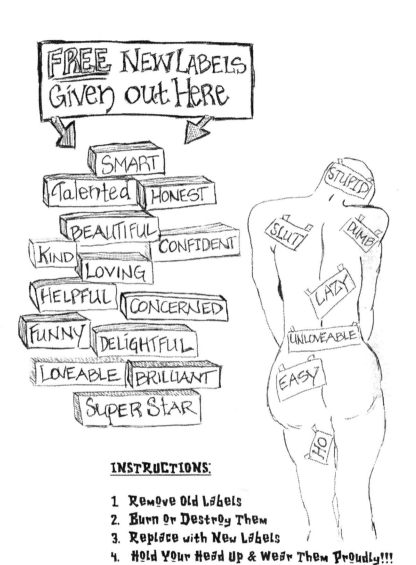

CHAPTER FIVE

What A Man-Child Wants

I call him a man-child because he is not a boy, and yet not quite a man. Not a full grown one anyway, especially when it comes to maturity. He may be taller than your daddy and have a little hair on his face, but he could easily be a baby on the inside.

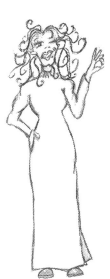

Since I'm not a man, (and wouldn't want to be one) I can only share with you what they have shared with me in terms of what a man (of any age) wants. This of course does not represent everything that he wants, but hopefully, you'll get the general idea.

A boy wants toys—the latest and the greatest. He wants to be loved and to have a stress free life. He wants someone to take care of his basic needs, feed him and give him time to play.

A man wants the same things. Toys, love, and a stress free life where his basic needs are being met, even if he's handling that himself. And he needs time, alone, to play with his toys his car, power tools, video games, or whatever. Added to the mix are his needs to release all of that physical tension that builds up, and that's usually accomplished through playing competitive sports, exercise and yep, you guessed it. Sex.

Men want to be respected and appreciated; and when they are, that's how they feel loved. They want you to pump them up, boost their egos and be their biggest cheerleaders.

A real man also feels the responsibility of taking care of all of his obligations, (even the little, crying, snotty-nose stinking ones). He wants to appear strong, courageous, and loyal. He wants to be the king of his castle, and the head of his household. Running things and holding it down.

Men want women who are independent and strong and who are financially stable in their own right. They want a woman who can bring something to the table other than her baggage and some other man's child. What they really want brought to the table is a home cooked meal, and fewer and fewer of them are finding that.

Because of testosterone, a male hormone, men are more interested in trying to figure stuff out so they are always taking stuff apart and then hopefully, eventually, putting it back together again. Women could really care less about that stuff—we'd rather go shopping and buy a new one anyway.

We are more interested in what other people are thinking and feeling. (And sometimes what they're wearing). Nothing will make a man want to flee from a room quicker than trying to get him to talk about his feelings, or asking him what he's thinking about. Men want to feel needed, but not from the endlessly needy. They want to be your hero, but they don't want to have to keep saving your behind over and over again.

They want someone they can be proud of and not someone they would be ashamed to be seen with in public. They definitely don't want someone who has been used so much it shows, or someone they could call Krispy Kreme who is, like their sign says, HOT NOW and ALWAYS OPEN. Unless of course that's all they want.

A man wants a woman who is so darned confident, that it looks sexy. They want us to share some of their interests, but also have some of our own. They want us to be a lady in the streets, but a freak in the sheets. Basically, they want us to represent.

They also want us to stop talking so much.

The guys in your age group are somewhere in between the boy and the man, and unfortunately, some of them will stay there. Forever. There are also days when they act like both a man and a baby boy at the same time, and trust me, some things never change. As you can see, the basic needs of men are pretty much the same.

There are many different types of men. I wouldn't say they were like snowflakes though. There are some that are just alike. Some of them blame women or everyone else in their lives for their mistakes, and that practice started with the very first man.

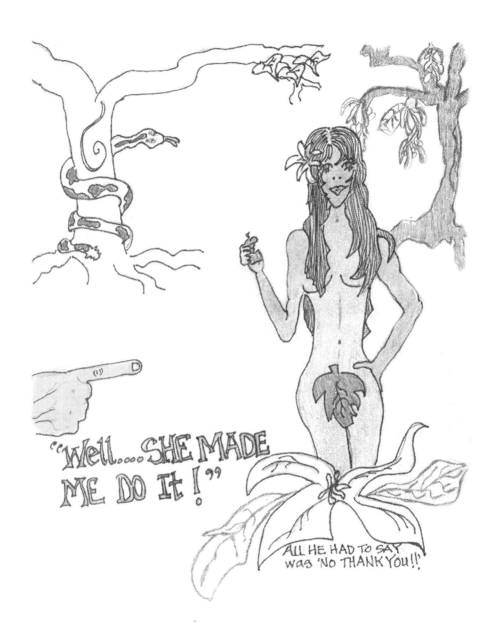

When God asked him if he'd eaten from the tree he'd been instructed not to eat from, Adam's reply was classic. "The woman you put here with me gave me some fruit from the tree and I ate it" (Genesis 3:12) I guess the word "No" hadn't been invented yet, or maybe the thought to refuse Eve never occurred to him. Anyway, he wasn't strong enough to resist, and men have been blaming us ever since.

Then there are men who would fight to the death for their honor (or yours) and take full responsibility for any wrongdoing even if they didn't do anything wrong. Strong, courageous, types that women want to be with and men want to be like. And then there are men that fall between those two extremes.

The bottom line is no matter how much we say they all seem alike, (especially when we're really mad at one of them) there are all types of men. But the basic core issues and characteristics of a man are pretty much universal and instinctive—meaning, it just comes naturally. There are two basic types that I will cover so you can get the general idea.

The Man as the Hunter

From the beginning of time, men were the hunters and the gatherers. Even Adam had to fend for himself after he'd disappointed God and was banished from the Garden of Eden "to work the ground from which he was taken" (Genesis 3:23).

The men left the comfort of their huts or caves for days at a time to hunt for food and provide for their families. Think about the image of the "caveman" or any primitive being. That's what he did, because that's all he knew. The writing was on the wall (so to speak), and he saw drawings of men hunting and spearing animals on the walls of his cave, and saw his father and the other male members of his tribe doing it as well. They usually did it alone. If they went out in packs, each hunter was responsible for his own kill.

The women, however, gathered together while washing or preparing meals, and knowing us, used the time to share their stories and the drama that was going on in their caves. Men were the lonely hunters. Women were just doing what we do.

After the kill, they would bring the animal back home, skin it and share it with their family. What they didn't eat, they used for other things.

They used the fur for coats and boots, the skins for clothing, blankets and drums, and the bones for weapons or jewelry.

In other words, they used what they had hunted until it was all used up. Whatever was left, and it usually wasn't much, was then thrown away.

Can you see where I'm going here?

Today, not much has changed. Except of course the hunting, killing and skinning of the animals has already been done for them. Now all they need to do is just hunt for a job in order to pay for the stuff.

A man today would probably pass out if you told him to skin an animal and make a coat and some shoes out of it. And then wear them. Girl, please. He'd rather throw himself down onto a very sharp object and then jump into a pool of alcohol. And it's "homemade" too! Men today would really be an endangered species.

But this easier way for men doesn't change the fact that his desire to hunt and gather (basically pursue and catch you) has not gone away. It's in their nature and it's in his blood. He couldn't help it even if he wanted to.

Most men will tell you honestly, that it is in the pursuit of the prey that is the biggest thrill for them. It's the art of the hunt, testing his skills and abilities (aka his manhood) that make him feel alive. Being crafty and outsmarting his intended target and then getting it gives them quite a rush!

Think about the men in your life who may hunt rabbit, deer, birds or women. Once they have captured (and killed) their prey, what do most do? Well, after they poke out their chest, pound on it with both fists, and let out a manly call of the wild, they bring a piece of it home and hang it on their walls to display their prize (except for the women of course).

It's all over for them. The thrill is gone. And they have evidence of their great skills, the proof is right there on the wall, only not a mere drawing this time. They have a constant reminder of what a great thrill the victory of their capture was and what a wonderful hunter they are.

That is until the next season or it's time to hunt again. Or a new girl shows up. Once the hunt is over and they have captured you (and maybe killed your spirit) they will be ready to move on. They will use all of you they need, for whatever their needs are at the time—attention, popularity, ego boost, or whatever—(hopefully not your bones for anything though), and then they will throw away what's left. And that is exactly how it will feel to you. Hunted, caught, picked apart, used and then discarded.

To continue to go after something they already have would be like shooting the mounted head that's already on the wall. Where's the fun in that? It doesn't prove what a master hunter they are, and that's what they need others to see. That's not a challenge for them and men need challenges. That's why they go out to look for a new thrill.

And you, sweetie, are left "hanging around" like another captured prize, trying to figure out what happened and why things are so different now. You are useless now except to prove that he caught you. Or at least a piece of you. That is if he hasn't thrown you away already.

He may keep you around during the off-season, blow the dust off of you every now and then when he needs to show you off to his friends or needs to use you up some more.

He knows you will always be hanging around, but can't seem to understand why you keep trying to come back to life, why you can't just hang there and accept your place. He caught you, game over and you should be happy about that. I don't think so!

What he's also captured is a piece of you. And you, in turn, will spend years trying to get it back. And then more years in therapy when you find out you can never get it back.

This, you can almost put money on. He is always going to be looking for the one that got away. The one who outsmarted him that he couldn't catch. The one who gave chase and made the whole thing more interesting and more challenging. The one that made him up his game and be more creative in his pursuit.

That's the one he'll dream of and desire and won't be able to get out of his mind. That's the one he'll remember forever and the one who he will fantasize about having. Not the one standing still with a bulls eye on their back. Or the one that's chasing him through the trees.

Besides wanting a woman who is independent, you know, has her stuff together, knows what she wants in life, and so on, what men are really looking for, although most won't openly admit it, is someone they can actively pursue. If you appear too easy, they will quickly lose interest.

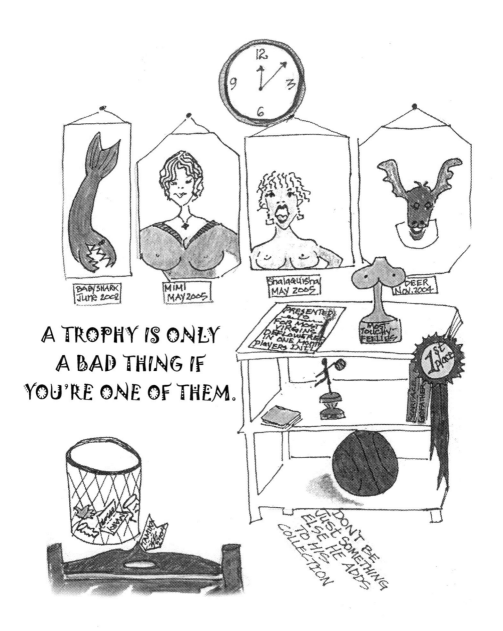

A TROPHY IS ONLY
A BAD THING IF
YOU'RE ONE OF THEM.

Be a challenge. Be the elusive one who always gets away and can't be captured. Make him work for what he wants. You'll be the one they talk about, long for and desire. They may even make it a competition thing because they want to be considered the greatest hunter of them all, the one who finally brings you down. You could even be a legend, like Big Foot. Everyone will know you exist, but no one can ever trap you, and they certainly aren't going to bring you down.

Besides, it's much more fun to drive him wild trying to figure out what he has to do to get you! The longer it takes the better it is for you. If he gives up too soon, that's a sign of weakness, and that is one thing for sure you want to know about a man from jump street. A weak man will never make it in the jungle, and life can be like that some times.

The Man as the Hero

How he'd love to have super powers like Mega-Strength, or X-ray eyes (to see through your clothes of course). If he could fly he'd be dangerous. Most little boys don their capes, either real or imagined, and pretend to save the world, or at least a lady in distress.

They practice various ways in which they gloriously die, clutching their hearts and gasping for one last breath. Either standing up to the bad guy, or being the baddest of them all, the end result is a fight to the death. And they die mightily and heroically with their boots on.

Women were made to give life and men were made to give theirs up. (For a noble cause, of course.)

Their fear is that they will not be mourned for as deeply as they hoped they would be, or honored and appreciated in a way that would be fitting for the heroic deed they'd done.

Heroes come in all forms, not just in battle or possessing super powers. They could dream of scoring the winning touchdown or making the final breathtaking shot right at the buzzer to lead their team to victory.

Men want to be admired and applauded for their skills, hoisted on the shoulders of their teammates and carried through the cheering and adoring crowd that's chanting out their name. It's not always enough to just win. They want to be the ones that make it happen. A statement worth repeating. The man wants to be the one that makes things happen. Super hero's don't need sidekicks. Batman didn't need Robin. A lot of times he just got in the way. They don't need your help to save you—you're doing enough already.

They don't want to do what every body else is doing, or have what everyone else has. Or has had. They have to succeed beyond the ordinary. The hero has to do better, and have better. He must succeed where others have failed.

He wants to feel worthy enough to be the one to save you from the other guy, a life of loneliness, or even from your own self. This is not to say that you should let every guy feel like a hero and come to your rescue and have you though. A lot of men are just perpetrating (pretending big time) as a hero to win you over and are not really in touch with the real hero that lives inside of them.

With time, and a clear understanding of who you are, you'll be able to spot the one that will be the hero for you. And you won't need a magic decoder device to find him.

Some are happy being the hero in secret, and others tend to need fans to cheer them and praise them for what they do. It's pretty easy to figure out which is which.

Even if he is not a hero, he would love to feel like one. He's been dreaming about it since kindergarten. Men need to be appreciated for their willingness to sacrifice it all in a heroic deed, either real or imagined. This is how they know they are loved. They want to (and sometimes need to) be the one who saves the day.

Until you really need a hero, it helps if you remember this. If a guy sticks up for you when somebody is trying to put you on front street, has your back at a time of need, or comes to your rescue before you fall down a flight of stairs, he's just awakened the hero that resides in him. Take a minute to acknowledge that, and appreciate him for his efforts, no matter how great or small.

It will make his imaginary cape blow gently in the breeze behind him as he secretly beams with pride for accomplishing yet another heroic deed. And having someone notice that he did.

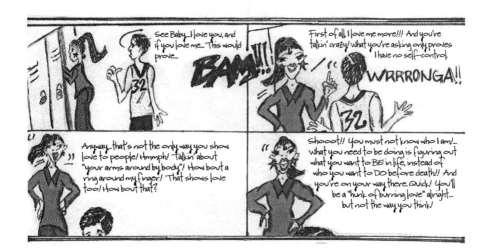

There is a LOT you can say!

CHAPTER SIX

He Says ... She Says

Sometimes, however adorable they may appear to be at the time, a man will say just about anything to try to get in between your legs or take you further than you are ready to go.

There may be occasions where your mind may not be functioning as well as it should because it's paying too much attention to what your raging hormones want to do. There is a delay from your brain communicating to your mouth to open and speak out an objection or something before it's too late...

Here are a few suggestions you may consider using when confronted with a request for sex to which you may not be prepared. Feel free to adjust them as necessary, and keep in mind, these should be used as a back-up alternative when your true feelings have been communicated, but don't appear to be heard.

If HE Says...   YOU Say...

"If you love me you will."   "If you love me you'll wait."

"I won't tell nobody."   "Since when do men keep that a secret?"

"You'll give me 'Blue Balls'.   "They'll go good with your Jeans."

"I thought we had something   "Me too. And not based on this."
special."

"Everybody's doing it."   "Allow me to re-introduce
                                    myself .... I'm not everybody. "
                                        Or
                                    "Let's dare to be different!"

"This will show me you   "We're too old for show and tell."
love me."

"It'll be real quick."

"And you're proud of that???"

Or

"but the memory will last my lifetime."

"I thought I was special to you."

"You are. And I'd like it to stay that way."

"You're such a tease."

"My bad."

"What are you waiting for?"

"What are you rushing for"

"Man, I thought you were a Woman!"

"I'm just not an easy one."

"You know you want some of this."

"I think you're confusing my wants with yours, and besides, "this" could kill me."

"I thought you were my Boo."

"Didn't know sex was part of that job description. You need to start taking other applications."

"What's it gonna take?"

"A lot more time and a ring on my finger."

"Girl, I'm gonna make you scream."

"A real scary movie could do that. Or did you mean **after** you leave me once you get some?"

"I can't wait to get some."

"I bet you could if you really tried."

"If you don't…·
Suck me - Touch it - Give me some… I'm gonna **EXPLODE!!!!**

"Wow, I'd hate to see you go, but it may be fun to watch."

My daughter and other teens I spoke with say guys these days "don't even have any game." Well actually those are my words, not theirs, but the point remains the same. Their approach is more direct, if, of course, you know what they mean.

"Do you wanna smash?"

"What's good for tonight?"

"What's good?"

"What are you on?"

These are just some of the examples of the things a guy may say as an invitation to sex. My first response, of course was disbelief, one at the lack of creativity, and secondly, that it could be so easy to get girls with just that and a nice smile.

Frankly, if some guy asked me "What are you on?" I would ask him the same question, because he'd have to be on something to think I would do anything with him with an invitation like that. What am I on? It wouldn't be him, that's for sure. Who comes up with these things anyway? The only thing you could say to questions like those above (or anything else as vague and meaningless) would be something like this:

"You're kidding right? Does that usually work for you? Do you really think that I would allow you to enter into a special, sacred and much desired place because you asked me a question that doesn't even make sense? Little Man, you need to go somewhere and get off of yourself, or, get off by yourself, and come back when you know how to talk to a woman."

If that doesn't work you can always try:

"You know I'd love to, but I'm not sure it's good for the babies. I'm having twins you know. Plus, I'm still waiting for these gigantic, pulsating, blister-looking things to go down a little bit, or at least stop oozing, bleeding and smelling so bad. Besides, the last guy I slept with is still in the hospital and I'm not sure if he lost one of his balls because of that, or not. Soon as I find out, I'll get back with you."

Make sure you wink and blow him a kiss before you walk away.

The more young ladies give in to this super casual sexual lifestyle, the more men will consider it the norm. It is not O.K. to be approached this way for anything, other than a casual greeting. Unless of course that person is a little off, or definitely off of his Medication.

It is demeaning and disrespectful and by responding in any kind of positive way, only encourages them to continue. If you can get away with a slap, do it. Maybe that will help him to snap out of it. Whatever you do, appear more disgusted than amused.

Tell him if he has some time you can give him tips on how to approach a young lady. They are doing what they think they are supposed to be doing, and if we don't help them, and tell them how it should be done, they may never know. We can provide a valuable community service to a generation of young men who will know what we want to hear, not that nonsense some of them are talking about.

We may never get back to the days when a woman hears:

"Baby, I want to share not only my life, but my innermost feelings with you, and explore our love in a number of intimate ways. I love your mind, your spirit and your body, and I can't wait for the day when we become as one. You are the perfect mate for my soul, My lighthouse through a stormy sea. I think of you every time my heart beats, because that's where you are. Where you are is where I want to be. You are a gift from God that I get to un-wrap everyday. Your wish is my will. My only desire is your happiness, and I live just to please you in every way a man can please and satisfy a woman. I give myself to you totally and completely. Just let me know when you're ready to receive me."

To have those days be a thing of the past is unfortunate for you young ladies. Mostly, because to be wanted for more than sex, being desired for our minds, our spirits, and who we are—that is the ultimate turn-on.

At the rate some of you may be going, you could be so depleted from giving away pieces of yourself that when someone finally feels that way about you, you don't believe it because it doesn't feel true. You may not feel worthy. And that screws everything up.

Lovemaking, really good lovemaking is an art. It's hard to create a masterpiece if your subject isn't around long enough to sketch him onto the canvas, or deep into your heart. It's even harder when the subjects keep changing and you have to keep starting over again.

To get to the beauty of what can be created, it requires certain steps, such as commitment, self-less-ness, and love. This is the ultimate high that you are seeking, and to use the experience to be for what God intended, to bring forth life.

The man (a real one anyway) should be about pleasing you (first) as well as himself. That's where being selfless comes in, where he's into your needs and desires before satisfying his own. If he really loves you, that will be his priority. You feel loved, cared for, whole, and everything's right with the world.

Casual sex is just that. Casual. There is no beauty in it, and it usually involves a few minutes of pleasure, mostly for him, and self-worth issues for you. There is no commitment, no love, and a lot of selfishness, which becomes more obvious during and after the sexual act. Afterwards, you feel empty and hollow. You are just being used, and there is something very wrong with that.

There will always be some 'after drama' to go through anyway, that's just the way it is. But it really doesn't have to be. Here's another chance for you to make a choice.

I mean think about it. Even if the guy was saying all that smooth stuff just to get in your pants, and as you know they will say anything, wouldn't hearing that be better than dealing with yourself and the after drama just because someone said "Do you wanna smash?" or said "let's get busy" or some other stupid, unromantic un-creative nonsense?

Girl, just say "no thank you" and keep steppin'. Tell them you have a vision in your mind of how it will be your very first time or the next time, and it will be on your honeymoon with your husband and at this point he couldn't even begin to come close. Especially with lines like that!

Tell him you are still taking applications for the one who will be worthy enough to have that honor & pleasure, but the criteria is not based on past experience... therefore references are not required. Tell him that so far you have not yet decided who the best man is for the job, but if he gets it, you'll be sure to let him know.

CHAPTER SEVEN

YOUR FIRST LOVE

Many of you will fall in and out of love many times in your life. Even married couples or couples in long relationships fall in and out of love with each other from time to time. I say that also because there can be those times when you think it's love and find out later that you were dead wrong. It happens to the best of us.

It sure can feel like love though. Feelings and emotions can be kind of tricky. Especially if those feelings are something new and different than we have experienced before. Love can be easily confused with many other emotions. And trust me, there are very few experts on the subject.

The falling "in" part is wonderful, enchanting, and beautiful. The falling "out" part can be very, very painful and sometimes, very, very ugly.

They say that you never forget your first love, and that statement is very true. The first time you fall in love can be beyond magical. How could you ever forget those initial "butterfly" feelings, pulsating body parts, and loud, quickly beating heart? And the breathlessness you feel whenever he comes near…

Not to mention that overwhelming feeling that you just have to be together every second, minute, and hour of each and every day! There's nothing like it in the world, and certainly not easy to forget.

That's why your first love, your very first love, should be you. Yeah, I know. This may sound crazy to you, but honestly, if you don't love yourself, no one else can or will. Truly, it all begins with you. And how you feel about yourself.

But first, you must realize who you are. Genesis 2:27 states:

So God created man in his own image, In the image of God he created him; Male and female, he created them.

God made both man and woman in his image and neither man nor woman is made more in the image of God than the other. No distinction is made between the two. They are both placed at the pinnacle [the highest point] of God's creation, and neither sex is held to a higher status than the other. Neither is depreciated. So why do we give men such power over us?

Maybe somehow we think it has something to do with the fact that we were formed from man's ribs (Genesis 2:22) but although we were taken from man, and made from his bone, that still does not lessen our role in God's plan.

He gave us one bone from men already, and we don't need to be trying to get another one. (If you know what I'm saying).

We were both created for the same thing. To worship and honor God. Man gives life to woman, (some men are still unhappy about that) and Women give life to the world. Each has it's own special privileges and neither one is better than the other. How could we be if were both made in his image?

To be made in God's image means we are reflections of His Glory by the way we live. It is our entire self that reflects the image of God and His character in our love, kindness, patience, forgiveness and faithfulness.

How could you not love someone who is made in the very likeness of someone with such wonderful qualities?

If he is the "King of Kings, and Lord of Lords," and He is your Father... what does that make you?

Exactly. The daughter of the King! Able to inherit the kingdom.

"Then the King will say to those on his right (those who are doing right and living right) 'Come, you who are blessed by my Father; take your inheritance, the Kingdom prepared for you since the creation of the World."   – Matthew 25:34

Not only did he make you in his own image, and equal to man, you are Royalty too!! Girl, you better Recognize!! We need to start acting like we know our heritage! And our birthright!

We need to begin to treat ourselves like the child of the most high that we are. There is absolutely no reason for you not to shine and be the reflection of God's Glory that he meant for you to be.

And since you never forget your first love, then you should always remember yourself, who you really are, and whose image you are reflecting!

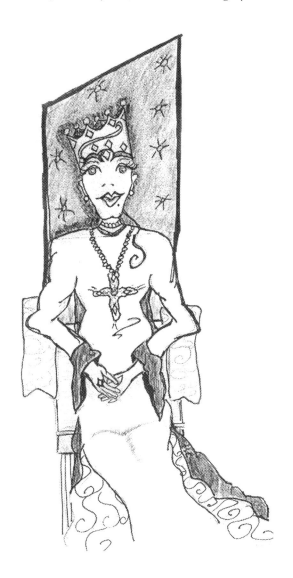

QUICK EXERCISE....

Oh come on. It won't take long. Grab a pen and a piece of paper. Quickly list 10 things that you love and adore about yourself. Why does that seem hard or funny? I bet if I said list all of the things you hate about yourself, you may need more paper. That's a shame.

When the list of things you love about yourself is much longer then the things you don't, you're on the right track. The love affair has begun.

When that list can be summed up in just one word—EVERYTHING—then look out world!!! A self-confident, self-assured woman will emerge, reflecting the image of who she really is, in all of her magnificent glory!

CHAPTER EIGHT

So You Really Think You're Ready?

At a certain point in our teenage years, our hormones start doing funny things, like bring on our menstrual cycle, start emerging little breast buds, and rounding out our hips. We may even get pimples and have an attitude for no apparent reason. We can almost see the changes taking place as our bodies begin to morph into these womanly shaped creatures. I have a friend who described this period as feeling as if she suddenly had these magical powers that made men, even grown ones, sit up and suddenly notice her. And she really liked it.

She no longer felt invisible to men. Suddenly, miraculously, (she thought) all these men were paying her so much attention! She could finally be seen, and she knew it had to do with her changing body. She felt the power of womanhood for the first time, and it felt good. She told me that she and a friend would often compete to see whose powers were the strongest or the most magical. Testing it to a limit, but not going all the way. She realized the danger in keeping that up.

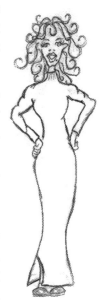

Our bodies go through transformations much like that of the metamorphosis that turns the caterpillar into a butterfly. Some of the stages aren't pretty. We feel awkward, far from attractive, and self-conscious. The end result, hopefully, is a beautiful butterfly emerges and flutters around in all her glory.

At this point, some of you may feel the need to spread things other than your wings. You feel this new body should be shared and these magical powers must be there for some reason. So many young ladies think at this point, they are ready for sexual relationships when truly, they are not. Now don't get angry with me; I know it's hard for someone to tell you that you are not ready. Especially when they don't even know you.

Just know that "being ready" has nothing to do with how long you've lived, or whether you think you are mature enough. Many of you have taken on responsibilities for yourselves, your siblings and other family members that give you the feeling of being mature, but maturity alone is not enough.

With more single parent homes, a lot of children are almost raising themselves. More and more of you are handling duties and responsibilities that a working or absent parent may not be able to do. Sometimes we feel as if we are grown because we are doing grown-up things.

Again, being grown isn't about the numbers. You don't turn a certain age, get sprinkled with magic dust, and Poof! you're a grown up. Surely we all know someone who should be grown, (you know, act like an adult) but they sure don't act like it, no matter how old they get. There are many different signs of maturity, but I will only cover a few.

Being mature is when you can talk about something other than boys, who said what about who, and how much you hate your life.

Maturity is when you can talk about, and dream about, what you love (other than boys), and what you want to do with your life during your short time here on earth. It's about trying to live your life with passion and purpose.

Maturity is taking total responsibility for yourself, including your mind and your body. It also includes taking care of the responsibilities of your home, and your finances. It is being accountable for the decisions you make, and acknowledging the mistakes made along the way.

It is paying the bills, bringing home the bacon, and frying it up in the pan. Maturity is about putting the needs and desires of everyone else in front of yours and what you want to do. And knowing when to say no so that people won't walk all over you in the process.

It's about obeying the rules even when no one else is around. It's when you know better, and then do better. In other words, it's about making the right decision when you know something you're about to do is wrong… whether anyone else sees you or not.

Being grown doesn't even guarantee success and the level of maturity needed to always make the right decisions when it comes to sexuality. Even grown-ups make poor decisions regarding sexual responsibility and the selection of partners. If you don't believe me, ask somebody. Find some adults you feel comfortable talking to and ask them if, in their adult life, they feel as if they have always made responsible choices regarding sexual behavior. You just might be surprised at their answers.

That's what people mean when they say you are not ready. They are not trying to put you down, insult you or even disrespect you. They just want to help a sister out.

There are so many feelings and emotions that go along with sexual intimacy outside of marriage: shame, fear, disappointment, resentment, humiliation, just to name a few. It makes you wonder that any of us are really truly "ready". One thing is for sure (although it probably disgusts you to acknowledge this): everyone, including your parents, has experienced the same exact feelings you have. All of them.

They had desires to want to kiss someone and be really, really close to them. They yearned to feel the nakedness of another body next to theirs, or at least see it! They had the butterfly fluttering around in the stomach feeling, the tingling, the throbbing and the wetness in their panties. (Boys usually have a different kind of wetness in their underwear known as "wet dreams").

Even our grandparents and all of our ancestors felt lust and desire - that's how we all got here. (Try to picture your grandparents not as you last remember, but in a more distant time when they were your age, or that of your parents. It helps.)

Desiring somebody, and wanting to be desired has always been around, from the beginning of time, and that is never going to change. Desire is not something that just started happening in time for you to experience it.

Being empowered to not easily act upon those desires is what has changed and truthfully, it seems like that is harder to control. Sex is everywhere. Music videos, TV, the internet, movies, etc. You almost get desensitized to it, and you just have to shake your head in amazement at what people will use sex to sell. Because it is everywhere, it is nearly impossible not to think about it. It's always right there in your face. It is when we act on those impulses and desires that get us into trouble.

Learning to control our feelings and put them in their place is also a sign of maturity, especially when you consider all of the risks that are involved. Sexual decision-making is a skill. It helps us control our sexuality not by stopping the feelings, but by putting them on a leash. A very short one.

It gives us the ability to pick a partner who respects us and our decisions. It also helps us avoid unwanted sexual outcomes, like pregnancy and sexually transmitted diseases. Not to mention avoiding the horrible way you'd feel about yourself once the act itself is over, he dogs you out, and then doesn't even call you anymore. Yes, it can even happen to you, especially if you have not developed the skills necessary to see that it doesn't.

Having knowledge alone isn't enough to stop or change risky behavior, but having it can give you what you need to make better decisions. Making responsible choices when it comes to your sexuality, or having the skills necessary to make the right decision, is not something you are born with. Instead, it is an acquired skill, and one that comes over time. It is not just something that comes to you when you think you are ready.

Part of maturity comes when you learn to take control. It's your body, and your life. You were the one put in charge of it. Don't let the media, the object of your affection, or your friends dictate to you when it's time to become sexually active.

If you do, you are handing the leash over to someone else and allowing them to lead you where you may not be ready to go. You are handing over your power and control. It's time to take it back.

Lust is a powerful spirit, but it too, can be controlled. God has given you the power to control it. You give it more power by giving in to those feelings and not keeping them in check, and telling them where they can go. The more you feed it by giving up control, the bigger it gets, and the harder it becomes to tame it. Stop feeding it. You are creating a monster!

You already have everything you need inside of you to do it. Feed the other one: The spirit of restraint. Soon that one will grow and take over, and you'll hardly have to worry about that worrisome lust anymore. Until it's time to. And then, it won't be lust; it will be love.

You have to find within yourself your own strength, power and self-worth. It starts by honoring yourself and your spirit. Just listen. Your spirit will tell you what it needs.

If it tells you that you need that cutie-pie you've had your eyes on, then that's not your spirit, that is your lust. Listen closer, and in time you will hear what your spirit is really telling you: "Love yourself, honor yourself, and treat yourself with dignity and respect."

WHY ASK WHY? Take the Test and Find Out.

Here's what you do... Let's say you think you've found someone you would like to share yourself with. I use the word share, because they will be taking a piece of you with them in a "to go" box as I've explained earlier.

If you really think that you may be ready, then give yourself the "Why?" test. It's where you continue to ask yourself "why?" after each and every statement you make in an effort to justify your decision that he is worthy of this gift. It's best to do this with a true friend because we can't always trust ourselves enough to get to the end of the test.

Have them keeping asking "why?" over and over, until eventually you will get around to the point where your bottom line reasoning for wanting it will point out how meaningless and shallow your desires to do it will be. They should keep asking the question until you eventually talk yourself out of it.

For example:

Girl, I think I'm gonna go on and let Wakeem get some.

Why?

I think I'm ready.

Why?

I wanna know what it feels like.

Why?

Because.

Why?

I just do. Besides I like him.

Why?

He's Cute.

"He's cute" is certainly not a reason worth giving yourself to someone for. In other words, "He's worthy because of the way he looks?" Is that your only criteria? You would actually allow someone to take you through all of the drama and unnecessary changes you will certainly go through because you like what you see?

We see cute stuff all the time. Hanging up in store windows, or strolling through the mall. It doesn't mean we have to bring them home!

I mean, I'm not saying that he has to prove himself worthy by running into a burning building and rescue your behind, or anything like that. I mean is he someone that could go from zero to hero if put to the challenge? And if you don't know, then you don't know enough about him to even give him your number. Just like you, it's what's on the inside that really counts.

Keep asking "why?" until you get to the core issue of why you really want to in the first place. "I just need someone to love me."

"I am extremely insecure and maybe this will help." "It feels good to be wanted." "I'm mad at my mother". "I'm tired of people treating me like a child." "I don't want to be the last one who hasn't". "I love him."

Whatever the reason you end up stating at the end of the "Why?" Test, the answer to the question should really be: "I hate myself so much that I am going to add humiliation and shame to the list of bad feelings I already have about myself so I'll treat my body exactly the way I feel. Like invisible, worthless, nothing."

Instead of hooking up with Wakeem, you should spend a little time with yourself and figure out what's going on there, and why you think so little of who you are.

Being with a guy, putting him in the middle of all that craziness and drama really isn't fair to him either, when you think about it. They already think we're crazy. Try blaming him for all of your problems because you let him get into your panties. That's a sure way to scare a brother off.

Then add "stalker" to your list of other things you don't love about yourself, because we tend to turn into one trying to figure out what went wrong.

Get your own issues straightened out before bringing someone else to the party. After all, he's not coming alone. He's bringing his buddies "ego" and "issues" with him.

When you're really ready to show up, then represent with your girls, dignity, confidence and control. Then the party will be a lot more fun for all of you.

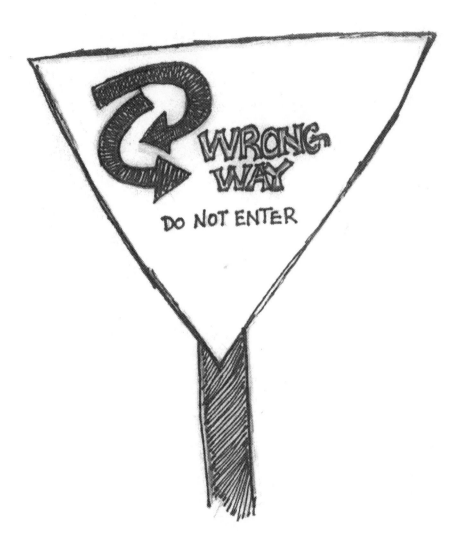

CHAPTER NINE

When Things Go Wrong, Don't Go With Them

There are times, however, when we become weak. That too, is normal. We let the excitement and these strange feelings get the best of us. Lust is whispering in our ear. It's like we go into a trance… a dream state.

Then we realize. "Uh oh. I've gone too far. I can't turn back now." The truth of the matter is, yes, you can. It is never too late to turn it around at any point as soon as you decide you don't want to go any further.

Even if you're as naked as the moment you were born, all he's wearing is a condom, and the moment of entry is about to begin, it's still not too late. I don't recommend or advise ever getting this close, however, but this is just so you'll know.

"No" means no, and "stop" always means stop no matter where you are on the road. Say it like you mean it, and run like the wind if you have to. But it's never too late to change your mind. Never.

The best thing to do of course is try never to be in that situation. If you think you are weak in the area of resisting, now is not the time to test yourself. Test yourself on other things that will not have the potential to kill you, like resisting spreading a rumor that you know isn't true. Resist the urge to try to instigate a situation just to get something started; going after that third helping of pizza; or getting on your brothers or sisters nerves. Practice resisting things that won't have a negative emotional effect if you fail.

Don't knowingly put yourself in situations where you are extremely vulnerable. For instance, being with a guy alone someplace where he is your only ride home and you don't have money for a bus or another ride home. Avoid being in any situation where you don't have the upper hand.

Drugs and alcohol seriously effect not only our decision-making skills, but our reaction time as well. Never let your drink out of your sight, or out of your hand. Some men put things in your drinks that you can't see or taste, that make you pass out and make you pretty much like a zombie for 18 hours or so.

They do this so they can repeatedly rape and sodomize you (put things like their penis or other objects in your body cavities like your vagina, mouth or behind) over and over again. And invite their friends.

Therefore, you should stay away from drugs, alcohol or anyone using them, so that your mind will remain clear and you are not under the influence of anything except the power of your own will.

Sometimes, though, we fail in our attempts to do the right thing. Occasionally, we slip up, have a brain fart, and our temporary emotions get the best of us. We feel that we are just too hot and bothered to resist the temptation. "Oh my God... It feels so good!" you think. So you give in to the moment.

Failure is not measuring up, not making the grade. It is the opposite of success. We also fail sometimes when we just give up. If we think something is too hard (and I don't mean it in that way) or won't come out the way we want, we just give up even trying.

But remember, failure is part of Life. It's that thing we do that hopefully teaches us not to do the same dumb thing all over again. And again, and again. Try to learn the lesson from your mistakes so you won't have to re-visit them in the future. You will keep repeating the same mistakes until you get it. They will just have different names and come in different packages.

You don't have to be stupid though. That's different. Being stupid is when you know something you're doing is wrong or will have a negative outcome, and you do it anyway. Sometimes we can be stupid from a lack of knowledge. When you have the knowledge or information and you fail to use it, or think that it applies to everyone except you, then you're just being stupid. And you are better than that. Who wants to be thought of as being stupid anyway?

Failure may be an okay place to visit sometime, but you don't want to live there. Or in Stupidity either. Turn around and head back to success and leave wrong right where it belongs.

CHAPTER TEN

The First Time

First, a Word to my Abused Sisters:

Most of us can remember certain events in our lives and all of the feelings come back as if we were experiencing them again. Our first bike, first pet, first day of Middle School, our first crush. As time goes on you will have other "firsts": first boyfriend, true love, sexual encounter, and heartbreak.

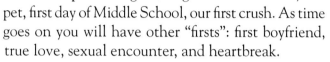

Unfortunately, many of you reading this have already had your first sexual encounter, but it was not your choice. A lot of young girls, far too many in fact, have been sexually abused or molested against their will by neighbors, family members, (so-called) friends, and even relatives. Sometimes even our very own parents are the ones causing the abuse.

I believe the latest statistics show that one out of every four women have been sexually abused, although the figure is probably a lot higher than that. Most cases are not reported and therefore do not become part of those statistics.

If you were to put a group of women together (of various ages) and the topic of sexual abuse came up, you'd probably find that more than half of those women could share stories of horror and abuse. In your classroom alone, there is probably more than one who feels ashamed of the secret she has been hiding and how it causes her to feel about her self.

Child molesters can be very sneaky, controlling, and manipulating, and could probably win awards for their acting abilities. They act like they are your friend. Someone you can trust and confide in. They may even have the trust of your parents. They may start off being playful and loving, and then suddenly, the relationship takes a turn that you didn't even see coming. How could you? It was inside of their sick head all the time, and you just got clued in!

They count on the fact that their intended target will not want to hurt or disappoint them by rejecting their advances. They also count on the fact that the object of their "affection" (although it is clearly not affection at all) will feel so bad that she didn't see it coming, that she will blame herself for being in that position in first place, and won't tell a single soul. He counts on the fact that her shame will keep her silent. That's all part of the master plan.

With others, it's just plain rape. A sudden violent, forced sexual assault on women against their will. Whether they know the guy or not, and most times they do. Often, women are raped by the men they are dating or seeing at the time. That's why they call it "date rape." If a woman is not ready and the man forces the issue - that's sexual assault and it's a crime. They take what they want when they want it, and the only thing they don't take is "NO" for an answer.

Whether you know the guy or he's a total stranger, forcing you to perform a sexual act against your will is a criminal act and should be reported. Maybe you thought you even liked the guy (before the act of course). If he can do that, clearly he has no respect for you, and is someone you should avoid at all costs.

Even exposure to sexual images (like magazines or movies) at a young or inappropriate age is also considered sexual abuse. Whether you are touched, or violated in any way, anyone who shows his or her body parts to you (on purpose, for the thrill it may give to them) may be a sexual predator and should also be exposed in an effort to stop that behavior. Such an act may make some girls more prone to curiosity about sex before their minds are ready or even capable of handling all that comes along with it.

Although a situation like those just described may have been a part of your past, it does not have to be a constant part of your future. You may not have had a choice with whom to lose your innocence or virginity to, but you can now choose abstinence (avoiding sexual relations) as a path away from promiscuity, (having casual sex with many people) which often follows such a traumatic event. Two things you must remember:

1. It was not your fault, and

2. You can try to stop the madness.

Most young girls feel that in some way they brought on the unwanted attack because of something they said, did, or didn't say or do. Others feel as if they got what they deserved because someone told them so.

Know this. Any person who willfully, deliberately and selfishly takes away a persons innocence for their own perverted needs is not even human for real. That may seem harsh, but that's opinion, and everybody's entitled to one.

Humans have feelings. They have emotions and the ability to tell right from wrong. Most predators (those animals that rob the innocence from their victims) that I speak of, usually don't even feel bad for what they've done. Part of which is to leave behind them a trail of hurt, shame, humiliation, pain and despair that at times seems unbearable, let alone unspeakable.

If I am talking to you, then I beg of you, find someone to talk to. If they don't believe you (as is often the case) tell someone else. Keep telling someone until someone hears you. And believes you.

Hopefully, this will stop the madness and the maniac creating it. Maybe this predator can be found out and locked up so this won't have to happen to anyone else. Find the power within you to speak up for your wounded self. Find your voice and use it to keep someone else from feeling the way that you do.

At a time when all control seems lost, find the courage within you to take enough control to see that this pervert doesn't do this to anyone else. Don't continue to give him power through your silence. Try to get some of your control back by using the power of your voice to expose him for what he is, and what he's done. You have control over whether he continues to abuse you or others. It's never too late to stop him.

Whatever you do, don't let what happened to you prevent you from hearing your own voice when it comes to making future sexual decisions that will be your choice.

Don't let that experience determine what choices you make in the future, especially in the area of sexual partners, or how you choose them.

Don't let negative thoughts about yourself based on that experience lead you to other negative experiences. Or down other dark alleys. Become your own light in the darkness, and see your way out.

In other words, don't blame yourself and then keep on punishing yourself by getting involved in relationships that keep making you feel bad about who you are. Or feel even worse about what was done to you.

You don't have to keep giving the abuser power over you when it comes to future decisions you make regarding your sexual behavior. Take that power back! You can control your life from here by making choices that show you still have value. No matter what he did, or how he did it. You are still a valuable human being! And you are also a survivor!

He's taken so much from you already. Don't let him take your value too! Besides, it's yours if you own it, and you already do! Wear it proudly. Just remember who you are and where you came from.

You are definitely not alone out there, although it feels that way at times. Seek professional help if you need it, and you most certainly do. Your pastor, a school counselor or school nurse, social worker, or any trained professional should be able to refer you to someone to get the help you need to start the healing process.

You could join a support group for women who have been victims of abuse, or you could even start one! It may help you to know that there are many others who can feel your pain, or even tell your story as their own.

Your innocence was stolen from you either by force or by trickery, and either way, stealing of any kind is a criminal act. Victims shouldn't be the only ones that are punished. Find your voice, girl!!! Lock him up so he can get a taste of what he did to you where he's going. I bet it won't be so much fun for him when he's on the receiving end!

Your First Time as a Willing Participant

With that said, let's try to explore the mystery of the intended First Time experience. I could almost guarantee you that it will not be the experience you expected. Unless, of course, it was a well-planned, well thought out experience with someone you really love, who really loves you back.

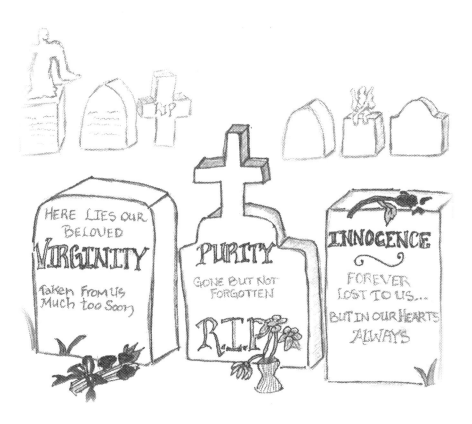

DON'T LET THEM DIE TOO SOON!

LET THEM LIVE LONG.... AND PROSPER

There are several important things that you must to remember. The first, and most important, is that afterwards, you will never, ever, be the same again.

Ever.

You will enter the point of no return, and no matter how much you practice abstinence, a virgin is something you can never be again. It is a step that once taken, will forever change who you are.

Your innocence is dead. Since it has been with you your whole entire life, you will miss it when it's gone. You will mourn the loss of it as you would a dear sweet friend.

Most young women don't quite understand the magnitude of taking this step. In fact, too many of you may rush into it for all the wrong reasons. Studies show that teenagers, especially black teens, are more likely to have intercourse for the first time out of curiosity about sex than for passion or even love.

What's up with that?

Don't let curiosity kill you or your cat! If there are things you are curious about, ask questions. Go to the library and do research on the subject. Gain knowledge and information. Resist the urge to transform what and who you are because you want to know what something is like or what something feels like.

The first time, more than likely, will be a big disappointment and not at all what you might expect. In fact, it could be one of the biggest disappointments of your life. (Up to that point).

Another important thing to remember is that the incident, that First Time experience, will be on constant instant replay mode throughout the rest of your entire life. No joke. Every now and then, something or someone will remind you of that experience and it will all come back. How it was, where it was and how you felt.

Wouldn't you want that memory to be a good one? One that made you smile or blush, instead of one that made you want to dig a hole just deep enough to stick your head in?

How would you like to re-live a moment over and over for all times that was a quick, unplanned disaster that was humiliating and regretful?

Maybe he was your first heartbreak as well. What if you didn't even really know his name or even what ever became of him? He's gone and a piece of you is gone with him. What if you found out he'd died from AIDS?

I met a woman who shared her First Time experience with me, and I could see clearly that she was still haunted by it. She said that it had occurred on the bathroom floor in a public restroom, in one of the stalls. Although it was not the romantic encounter she had always envisioned, she said that she went along because she got temporarily caught up in the moment, and was afraid to back out because she didn't want to lose the guy.

A few awkward moments later, as they got up and prepared to leave, they noticed that someone hadn't even bothered to flush the toilet. She couldn't get that particular image out of her head, and to this day, says she still feels like that piece of poop that was floating around in the toilet. And can still feel the cold tiles on her neck and shoulders.

To this day, she still has a problem using public restrooms, and whenever she must, memories of that night fill her with regret all over again. And what ever happened to that guy that she was so afraid of losing?

She said that after that night, she could never even look at him bcause of shame and disgust. She was ashamed that she'd allowed herself to be put in that kind of situation, and disgusted that someone she thought cared about her could even put her there. The truly hurtful part was that he made no effort to figure out why they'd stopped talking, and didn't even seem to care one way or another.

That experience gave her a room in the Heartbreak Hotel and every time she is reminded of it she unlocks the door and mentally checks back in.

Everything comes back. The smells, the sounds, the feelings. Wouldn't it be better to have a moment to re-live that was one whose very memory of it brings about those same fluttery feelings and racing heart that you felt when it happened?

Wouldn't you want your mind to unlock a door that was full of warmth and joy instead of emptiness and pain? You are the key. Besides, the Heartbreak Hotel is already filled to capacity... find another room elsewhere.

I'm just saying. It's your choice how you want to keep remembering that moment. And you will. So chose wisely with forethought in mind. Plan it out for how you'd like for it to happen, a scenario worthy of your most precious gift. You deserve more than some quickie in a place where you have no business being, one that was not designed for a sexual act, or one not worthy of your heritage.

Anyone who tries to put you in that position, (bathroom stall, closet, locker room, kitchen floor, or wherever) only cares about one thing. And you are not it. You know you deserve better. If you don't give in, he'll soon know it too!

The best way, I think, is to be able to tell the story to your children, as you recall the special way you felt anticipating the experience with someone you truly loved. You laugh quickly as you remember how funny it was as you nervously tried to figure it all out together.

The awkwardness of it all and literally exposing all of who you are to someone for the first time, remembering how nervous and unsure you both were at exactly what to do, and just how you were supposed to do it. And the excitement of finally discovering what it was all about. Being so close to someone you could really trust.

And recalling the beauty of how special it was to share yourself with someone that was worthy and deserved the gift they were about to be given. Because they understood how special and priceless it was and because you knew you could trust him to take special care of it. At that moment, that man, also smiling now from the memory, reaches over and gently squeezes your hand as you tell the story.

It may sound like a fairy tale, but it does not have to be one. You say it doesn't happen that way anymore, and I say it can. I guess we're both right. If you believe that it can't happen then it won't. The opposite is equally true.

Make your first time unique and one you don't mind remembering. Convince yourself that you deserve nothing but the best. Remember who you are, and the value of what you have. Be selective. Be patient. And be safe.

By the way, one more thing on the subject.. ..

THERE IS POWER IN PURITY!

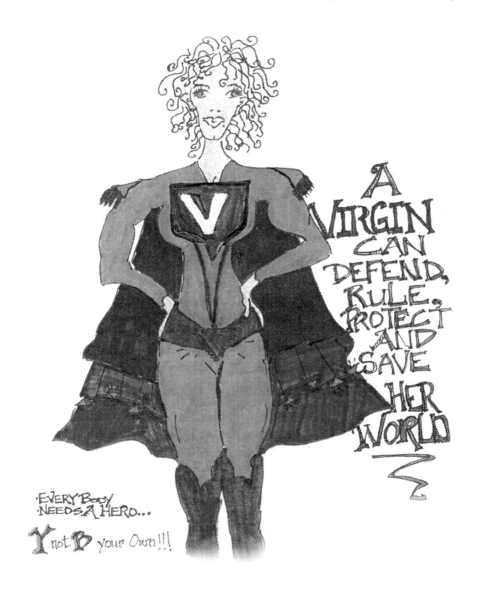

A VIRGIN CAN DEFEND, RULE, PROTECT AND SAVE HER WORLD

EVERYBODY NEEDS A HERO...

Y not B your Own!!!

LADIES... HELP YOUR SISTERS OUT - PLEASE COME CORRECT!

There is this tendency for some of you, who are no longer virgins, to really stretch the truth about sex or your sexual experiences. A lot of young ladies put down others as a result of their lack of experience in the sexual arena. They make fun of those who are or would like to remain virgins, or make them feel like they are missing out by not 'putting out'. They talk about it all the time, and really make it seem greater and way more exciting than it actually may have been.

Aside from the fact that misery loves company, what those women may be trying to do is to make you more like them (experienced) even though they may have regrets—they don't want others to know their shame and disappointment. Certainly, they don't want to feel this way alone.

Ladies, Please Speak the Truth! Tell your sisters how it really was, how you really felt, and how you really wish you could have waited.

Tell them to hold on to their innocence as long as they can, and celebrate it with them (if you are woman enough). I could almost guarantee you that you will be a better woman for it.

Saving the spirit of another woman by not allowing her to repeat the same mistakes you made could be one of the greatest contributions you could make to your sisters in the struggle.

You may never know how many lives you could actually save by speaking the truth, and coming correct. Although you may not know how you would be blessed for that, just know that the blessings will be coming.

Besides, the young woman whose very life you could save (by not rushing into a sexual relationship based on a lie that she was told by you, having unprotected sex, and then contracting an incurable disease) may be the one who discovers a cure for AIDS. Or Cancer. You never know what impact you can have on the lives of others, simply by speaking nothing but the truth. Especially in an area where so many lives are ended needlessly by trying to follow the crowd.

Be a blessing. Dare to be different! Be honest and be blessed!

CHAPTER ELEVEN

And BABY Makes OOPS...

For these young men making babies, you can believe that unless they are a rare species, fatherhood will be much like their sexual experience. Amusing, temporarily satisfying, and very easy to walk away from.

They will be unattached to you and the child because they do not have the same level of commitment that you have. There is no emotional connection to you and he will, therefore, probably not have one for your baby either. They will soon be off looking for yet another hole to fill, and will appear clueless as to why you are so devastated when things don't work out with the two of you.

He'll say you're trippin' and he will be right. What did you expect? He'll say he thought you wanted it too, but won't realize that what you wanted were two entirely different things.

If you are 'doing it' because it seems like everybody else is, then find other people doing other (positive) things for you to follow and imitate. Better yet, be a leader and not a follower. Encourage others to respect their bodies by not just giving them away for the asking. Dare to be different!

I know you're special, and hopefully you will get to the point where you believe you're special too. But with that said, what makes you the one that would be soooo special that things will be different for you than all the other girls before you?

If you give up the goodies just like all the other girls, how can you stand out as being any different from them? Try to be special in other ways, like being the one who refuses. That he will remember, and that will be what sets you apart from all of the others.

Having his baby will not give you the results you may be seeking, or bind you to him in the way you hope it will. In fact, it could have quite the total opposite effect:

You could be hated and despised for tricking him (that is what he will

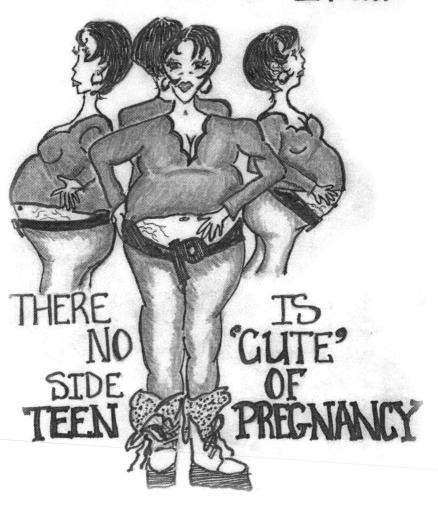

say, anyway) into having a baby. You will be called all sorts of names that you don't deserve, and then you'll have the added frustration of walking around looking like a whale, when all the other girls he's now talking to are wearing cute little outfits.

Then you become a BMW (Bitter Mad Woman) and you don't eeeeven recognize who you are your own self, and now you're bringing along someone else on the trip. And Baby Makes Oops... Two babies trying to raise one another.

Have you ever noticed the force of a magnet as it tries to connect with the refrigerator or another magnet? The same amount of force equally repels the magnet, and you can't get anywhere near it. No matter how hard you try, you cannot get them to ever connect.

Imagine that you and he are those magnets. That force that once attracted you together with a desire and longing you couldn't explain, let alone seem to control, has now flipped on the inside of him once he got what he wanted from you.

As such, it will make it impossible to want to be near you. No matter how hard you try, that force that drew you together is now keeping you apart. Not even a baby can fix that, in fact, it could be the baby that makes him flip in the first place. Thinking about everything involved in raising a child is certainly enough to make anyone flip. Especially when the baby's mother is a virtual stranger to you.

Wouldn't you rather be the magnet that draws him to you, rather than away?

Don't allow a child to be a constant reminder of how differently you both felt about the sexual act or each other at the time. Doing so will only set you up for a lifetime of trying to get him to be involved in his child's life. Or not. You deserve better, and so does an innocent child.

No child should begin his or her life unwanted by either or both of their parents. Or merely as a result of curiosity of what something will feel like. By no means should a child begin its life just to keep someone in yours.

I have to say this just for the record.

HAVING HIS BABY WILL NOT MAKE HIM LOVE YOU.

He may not even love the baby. He could have enough of them already. He could be enough of one already.

And really, just think about it logically for a minute. You would actually expect this guy, who feels like his whole life is ahead of him, to get a job (because he probably doesn't have one already) and take care of a child that he doesn't even want? From a sexual experience that wasn't even a relationship??? Why would you expect him to care about a baby when he doesn't even care about you for real? He only said he did and you really wanted to believe him.

Look At the Big Picture... The Whole Ugly Thing

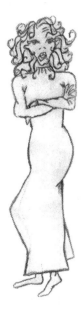

Should he have to pay for this life he's bringing? Absolutely. Will he? Probably not. Who picks up the tab? Who pays for the pre-natal care, the hospital bill, the food, the clothing and the shelter for this child? We all do. Our government through collecting taxes from its working people enables social programs to provide for these children whose parents aren't able. And if that doesn't bother you, then it should.

Should you be mad that he's not taking care of his child? Absolutely. Will your being mad make him be financially responsible? Absolutely not. It's not like you didn't know having sex could make a baby. You have a choice. Stop making these innocent babies and society pay for your few minutes of maybe a good time. We are "throw away" women making "throw away babies".

Why should it be okay for everyone in the state you are living in to financially support a child that came as a result of not being conceived through marriage, caught in a condom, or is here because "Yes" was said instead of "No".

If you can't see that making a baby and having everyone else—even total strangers who make responsible choices and take care of their own babies—take care of yours is wrong, then clearly you are not ready to be sexually active.

Sometimes, women get locked into a "generation" kinda thing. They think it's okay just because their mother did, their Aunties and even their grandmother may have relied on the assistance of the Government to care for their children, and they are just doing what everyone else in the family did. It's time to break that cycle. Assistance when you are down and out is one thing, but relying on it to care for your children is not providing them the opportunities to which they should be entitled. Especially when all you have to do is control your desires, or at the very least, use protection.

If you are grown enough to make a baby, then be grown enough to provide for it. Yourself. You know? I'm just saying. Yet another reason why you really should wait until marriage to have sex. The state is not your man and should not be the one to provide financially for your child. I'm sure this is going to make some of you angry, but I hope you keep reading because what I am saying is the truth, and sometimes the truth really hurts.

Why lock yourself into a system that is designed to keep you down? Designed to keep you from reaching your full potential? It is a system that is designed to lock you in and keep you in the lower class of society and sometimes forces you into illegal situations just to make ends meet. You are smarter than that. And you and the future generations deserve better than that. You can have a better life and it's based on the choices you make.

Let's be for real... unless he already loved you before, and not just said he did, but really, really, loved you, then why would he start now? If you don't love yourself, why should he? If you are giving yourself away so easily just for the asking, you are not expressing self-love, and that only opens the door for others not to love you too.

Some of you have a baby to get the love you seek, but you need to know that although your baby will love you, it's not the kind of love that you are actually seeking. You only think it is. In the beginning you do far more giving than receiving anyway. And it's a love that comes with a lot of responsibility... not the carefree, butterflies in the stomach, head in the clouds, music playing in the background kind of love that we are all trying to find. Just ask a young mother who already has one.

If it is love you seek, start first by giving it to yourself. That's where it has to begin anyway. Besides, wouldn't you want someone to love you because they choose to and not because they have to?

Some have babies because they think having one makes them a woman. Womanhood is not necessarily achieved automatically when you conceive or deliver a child. Especially if you are not able to completely provide for that child. There are no shortcuts to womanhood. If your parents, grandparents or the State are providing for you and your child, that doesn't make you a woman. That makes you a statistic. And you are so much more than that.

If you really care about the world in which you live, (as you really should) and you want to make a difference in it (as you really can), realize this. We can greatly decrease the number of angry, hostile, and worthless feeling people in the world by bringing babies here who came as a result of love through the commitment of marriage. Where both parents are ready, willing, and financially able to provide for all the needs of that child. Be that statistic instead.

Enough of the Big Picture... Just remember, making responsible choices is really what separates the women from the girls. Always make choices that honor your value and you're on the right track to woman-hood. Without the baby and diaper bag in tow!

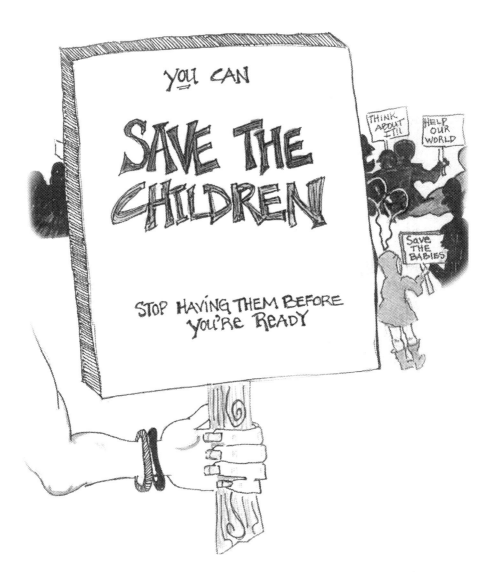

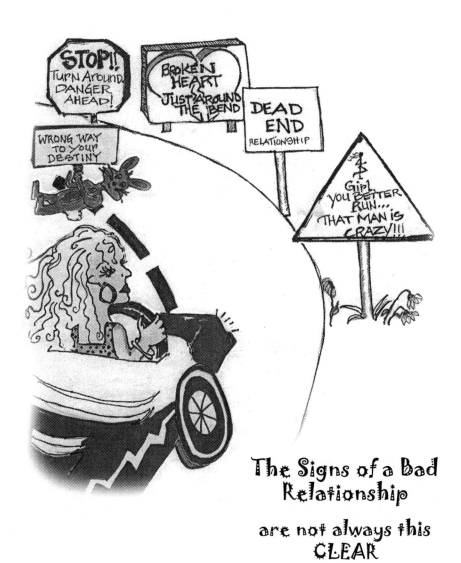

CHAPTER TWELVE

Signs of A Bad Relationship

Sometimes it's hard to tell if you are in a relationship that is not good for you, or one that could cause you harm. If you think that you could be in one, get out as soon as possible. If you are not sure, ask a parent, a friend, or someone you trust who has seen the two of you together, and see what they say. Talk to your Pastor, a school counselor or someone you trust, who can be honest with you about what they see.

Love can be a blinding thing, and what may be obvious to everyone around you may not be clear to you until it (or he) hits you in the head. If people are saying things to you about your relationship, or how this guy is keeping you away from your friends, take heed, and listen to what they are saying.

The best measure you have is what your gut and gut feelings are telling you. If you have an uneasy feeling, or something just doesn't feel right, pay very close attention to what you're feeling, because those feelings are never wrong.

Those feelings are called intuition, among other things; and its job is to protect us and keep us from harm. It is our internal alarm warning and alerting us of danger. Unfortunately, it doesn't come with flashing lights and sirens, but even still, those feelings should not be ignored. Under any circumstance.

Sometimes it could feel like goose-bumps and hairs standing up straight. Other times it could be a sudden and overwhelming feeling of darkness and doom. Sometimes, it could be just a little voice that says, "Hmmmm", or a whisper that says, "something isn't right." It could be a loud booming voice that says "Get Out Now!"

Don't ever try to excuse or justify the behavior of someone who is not treating you right, because frankly, there is no reason for anyone treating you badly. You are a Queen, and deserve to be treated like one.

The following list are not all the signs that indicate you could be in a dangerous or even fatal relationship, but I believe these are the most obvious. If you are experiencing any of these, get out of there as soon as possible. It could save your life.

WARNING SIGNS TO LOOK OUT FOR:

1. **If he seems too controlling.** Controlling what you wear, how you wear your hair, who you can talk to or hang out with, how you spend your time this is usually a sign of someone who wants to control every aspect of your life. Don't let them. This is not love. This is control.

2. **If he displays abusive behavior** or he shows a tendency towards violence, towards you or others, pushing, shoving, slapping or punching. Even if it starts off playful, it could graduate into something more. Love does not hurt. (Not physically, especially) If he hits you, and tells you he loves you, clearly he's confused about what love is. **YOU CAN NOT FIX HIM.** Leave that to a trained professional. No one should put their hands on you for any reason! If he does, walk away quickly and never look back.

3. **If he constantly puts you down,** talks about you to humiliate you and tries to make you feel worthless beware! Does he call you names and try to make you feel dumb? Or that you are not worthy enough to be with him? This is part of his whole manipulation plan to make you feel so bad that you don't feel worthy enough to be with anyone else. (If you are so bad, why does he want you?) Love edifies (lifts you up); it doesn't put you down. If he's treating you this way then you need to put him down.

4. **Is he always unavailable? Unless he wants sex?** Is he only nice to you when he needs something from you? He's a user and will continue to use you until you stop the madness. If he loved you he'd make time for you. He is not worthy of you or your time.

5. **Does he have all of your numbers (home/cell/etc.) but you don't have any or all of his?** Why do you think that is? Can he come to your house, but you are not allowed at his? Chances are he's already involved with someone else and you are just a little plaything on the side. Tell him you need someone who can be available when you need him; and if he's not the one, then find himself another playmate.

6. **Does he seem real secretive?** Does he keep a lot of things away from you basic things like his real name, where he was born, etc.? Unless he's undercover with the FBI (or maybe wanted by the FBI) that could be a sign that he could keep other things from you as well, like whether he's killed anyone before he met you.

Men tend to be on the quiet side and don't share nearly as much info as we do, or as we'd like for them to. But if it's general info that he's hiding, this should be a warning that he may be keeping something from you that could be dangerous. Intimacy and love are built on trust and it's hard to trust someone not willing to share themselves with you.

7. **If he hates his mother, disrespects women,** and doesn't seem to think too highly of our sex, there is nothing you can do to change his opinion. He will not treat you the way you deserve to be treated. He could even be hiding some deep, dark secret hatred towards women and may take it out on you.

8. **If he isolates you from your friends, family, or other people** and events and wants to keep you all to himself, girlfriend don't be flattered. Be very, very afraid. This is another example of a controlling man, and while you may think he loves you so much that he always wants to be with you, he is obsessed and is getting everyone else out of the way so no one can report you missing. These are usually the ones that say something like "If I can't have you no one else can" right before they murder you. Don't ever let any man keep you from your friends.

9. **If he ever threatens you or members of your family, believe him!** See him in that moment as the kind of man capable of carrying it out. Those are not the thoughts that a normal, sane individual would have. Just know that you are looking at crazy right there in your face. Know that the heart pounding quickly and loudly and the feeling of being light-headed and breathless all at the same time... that's not love, sweetie. That's fear.

Run like the wind no matter what kind of shoes you have on! Use your legs to get away while you still can.

If you see any of these traits in the guy you like, or that likes one of your friends, get out (or tell your friend to) quick, fast and in a hurry.

I mention them here because at times women (of all ages) confuse feelings of being controlled or feelings of fear with those of love. Don't confuse your emotions or let your emotions confuse you. The bible says in Jeremiah 17:9, "The heart is deceitful above all things, and desperately wicked: who can know it?" This means we cannot always trust what our heart is our feeling.

So to protect yourself, learn how to set boundaries for yourself, and don't let anyone cross them. It could save you from years of agony in an abusive relationship and could even save your life. And it's one that is certainly worth saving.

CHAPTER THIRTEEN

Helpful Hints for Better Relationships

Being a teenager or a young woman is hard enough, but being one nowadays is down right frightening. I honestly don't envy you and wouldn't trade places with you for a lifetime of youth and beauty. Since we have already examined some things to look out for to prevent getting involved in a bad relationship, here are a few things to consider regarding relationships that may help you find better ones as you journey into the wonderful world of womanhood.

QUALITY TIME

The best way to develop an intimate relationship with someone is to spend quality time with them. Secrets are shared, new interests and talents are discovered, and you get to see what kind of person they really are deep down on the inside, where it really counts. I'm talking about spending that quality time with your own self, because you can't truly be yourself when you meet someone if you don't even know who you are.

> **TIP:** One good way to find out more about your self is to keep a journal. You don't have to write in it daily, but a journal can be an excellent place to express yourself and to confide your private thoughts, dreams, or fears. It is also very enlightening to look back through the months or years and see who and what you were interested in at the time, where your head was, and how clearly you have grown since then.

BRING OUT YOUR BEST

The best way to tell if a relationship you're in will enrich your life or rob you of it is this. Ask yourself these questions: Does it bring out the best in you and what you have to offer? Are you a better person because he is in your life? Have some positive things come about either because of him or your relationship with him? Is he someone you admire and does he inspire you to do or be better in some way?

If your answer to all of these questions is yes, then you're probably not in a toxic relationship. If there are more negative things that came about in your relationship, then maybe that one positive thing about him shouldn't even be counted. For instance, if he smacks you around a bit, or puts you down constantly, then who cares that he tells you to look pretty. You won't for long! If he doesn't bring out your best or bring out the best in you, then you shouldn't even be wasting your time. Real love or a good relationship should make you better because of it.

MAKE A NEW FRIEND

Introduce yourself to confidence. It's hard sometimes to display a positive self-image because we don't often have one. There are so many things that we dislike about ourselves, that all we manage to show others is our obvious lack of confidence.

Confidence is a firm belief in anyone or anything. Unfortunately, most of us are not confident about our abilities, our looks, and so many other things. In fact, the only thing we are firm about is the belief that we are really not sure of ourselves.

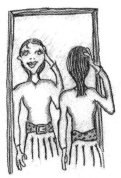

LEARN TO REALLY LOVE & ADMIRE THE PERSON STARING BACK AT YOU IN THE MIRROR

It's time you made a new friend named confidence, and in embracing that new relationship, a more self-assured 'you' will break through. Focus on those things you like about yourself, the talents you have and those things that make you unique and special. Believe in yourself and accentuate the positive focus on and promote those things that you are good at.

Once you become your friend instead of your own worst enemy, a new confidence will begin to shine through. In time, your head will be held a little higher, and your walk will become more pronounced, more sure of where you're going. Your entrance into a room will speak volumes without you ever saying a word. And that is how it should be.

When people believe in you it inspires you to do great things. Become a firm believer in yourself! Confidence is a great friend to have around, and if you become acquainted with it now, it can be your friend for life... Your own personal fan club. Every one of us deserves that.

A FRIEND INDEED

It is said that our friends are the family we choose for ourselves. Never underestimate the power of the relationship of a true 'sister-girl-friend'. It is our friends that can stay in our lives forever, through the joys, pains, and hurts of life, love and relationships. They can keep it real with you, cheer you, inspire you, and if you're lucky, love you even when no one else will.

To have a friendship that spans the years of marriages, births of children, and all other such milestones on the road of life-- to have someone with whom to share it all with is simply priceless. Connect. Do it sooner than later. You'll have many more memories to cherish between you.

Friendship is the gift you give yourself that keeps on giving. Seek one. Be one. A friend in troubled times, a friend in really good times. A friend in need. A friend indeed.

THE OTHER WOMEN

Pay close attention to the relationship a man has with his mother, his sisters, and other women in his life. If he loves and admires his mother, and treats other women respectfully, you can be sure you're in good hands. How a man treats his mother is usually a very good indication of how well you will be treated, or not. His relationship with her usually determines how he generally feels about and treats women.

Is he respectful and caring? Does he try to please her and seem to take good care of her? Does he speak of her in positive ways? Or does he seem to put her down and would appear to spit on her if the opportunity presented itsself? Does he consider his mother to be cold and manipulating, or loving and kind?

If you don't know what his relationship is like with his mother (or other women in his life), hold off on developing a relationship with him until you do. Find a man who adores his mother (but not to the point of being weird and creepy) and he is almost sure to adore you too.

KNOW YOUR PLACE

Once you have arrived at the place where you believe in yourself, know how valuable you are, and how much you have to offer, stay there. Your standards should rise up and meet you there. In other words, know what you want, and how you want to be treated, and don't allow anyone to treat you any less than that! For any reason. Period.

Do not compromise when it comes to your standards of acceptable and honorable behavior. Remember whose child you are (that of a King) and don't allow anyone to treat you any less than the way you deserve to be treated. Settle for nothing less than the best! After all, you deserve it!

CHAPTER FOURTEEN

Tips for Talking With Your Parents

Not quite sure how to talk to your parents or significant others? Here are some suggestions to get you started.

Timing is Everything

Timing is crucial to how you will be received. If your parent seems frazzled, or stressed out, the phone is ringing, the dog is barking, "what's for dinner?" is being considered, and siblings are trying to get their attention, then that may not be a good time to make your approach.

If, on the other hand, their lives always seem that way, just let them know that you would like to schedule a few minutes of their time. So they won't be alarmed or afraid, just let them know you have some questions you would like to ask, get their opinions on something, or let them know some things you may be going through.

Once they know that the police don't need to be called and no ambulance is necessary, they can relax a bit and make a mental note to get back with you. They will probably ask one of the following questions, so be prepared with your answer.

"Is everything all right?" "Are you in any trouble?" "Do I need to get my belt?" "Is it an emergency?" "What's it gonna cost me?"

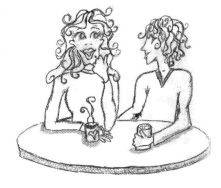

Reassure them that though not an emergency, you would like to talk to them soon, (before you lose your nerve) and that it's just about Maturing Stuff. They may be an adult, but sometimes you have to make the first move.

The Fear Factor

I'm talking about theirs, not yours. Parents are usually in denial or are extremely naive when it comes to what their children are doing. They sometimes fear the worst, and often don't ask questions for fear their suspicions will be true. Or even worse than they'd imagined.

They are also very afraid of appearing hypocritical--telling you not to do something that they may have done, or may still be doing.

Try to stay away from questions about what they did in the past and the discussion will be easier for both of you. Everyone makes mistakes, including your parents. Try not to be judgmental, and just remember, some things are better left unsaid.

Too Much Information (TMI)

Whatever you do, try not to shock them out of their shoes. There is a danger of giving too much information when just the basic facts will do. Take the following situations for instance, and see how each way can give you a totally different approach to and response from your parents.

The Situation: You are no longer a virgin, in fact you have been sexually active for about a year and have had two partners. Your parents are not aware of this. Last weekend, you attended a party and although alcohol was being served, you did not have any. However, you believe that someone may have put something in your can of soda while you were not watching, because you appeared to have blacked out and don't even remember how you got home. You have aches, pains, and soreness on certain areas of your body that you can't explain. You believe you may have been sexually violated (raped) by several guys at the party, because people are talking about it at school. You feel lonely, ashamed and afraid because you don't know what to do.

WRONG APPROACH

"Mom. We need to talk. I think some guys may have ran a train on me at that party last week. They didn't take my virginity or anything, but people at school are laughing and talking about it, and I don't know what to do."

96

Your mother will be stuck on the virginity part and may not concentrate initially on the situation at hand, because she's dealing with the shock that you have been sexually active. Her next thought may be that you were probably drinking and the sympathy that she should feel may take a while to surface.

Your parents' guilt for not being able to protect you may display itsself as anger or hostility instead of the compassion you may be seeking.

BETTER APPROACH

"Mom, I'm sorry we haven't talked more before now, but I think I may be in trouble and I really need your help. You were right about that party I went to, there was alcohol being served there, but I didn't have any because I know how you feel about that. I think someone may have put something in the soda I was drinking because there is a lot from that night that I don't remember. I believe I may have been raped because that's what some people are saying at school. I'm afraid, and I don't know what to do."

Although you have given more information here than in the first scenario, you kept the focus on the situation. I'm not suggesting keeping your sexual activity from your parent, I'm suggesting that at the initial introduction to this conversation, that info could be distracting. It will come up, maybe within the next few minutes, but to mention it at the onset may not be a good idea.

You have hinted that there is more to tell, shown responsibility by not drinking, and painted a picture that would help your parent focus their attention where it needs to be focused. Getting you help, (medical and otherwise) getting information, and getting the police involved if a crime had indeed been committed.

The Situation: You are 17 and still a virgin. You have been dating your boyfriend Tony for about 8 months, and you think you are ready to take your relationship to the next level. You love Tony and you want him to be the first one. What you don't want is to get pregnant, or a disease, so you approach your mom for guidance.

97

WRONG APPROACH

"Mom, I love Tony and he's my Boo. I'm ready for him to make me a woman, but I don't want a baby. Can you take me to get some pills or something? Oh yeah, and is it O.K. if we do it my room?"

Unless you want your Boo to see you toothless with your mother's hand print on your face, this is not the approach I would advise. And no, it's not okay to do it in your room!

BETTER APPROACH

"Tony and I have been dating for a while, and I think we really love each other. How will I know when I'm ready to take our relationship to another level? I'd like to talk about the different birth control methods that are out there to see which one works best. What do you suggest?"

Your mother, though no doubt shocked and taken back, will appreciate the fact that you are considering the act in a mature fashion and trying to get more info. She will also like the fact that you asked her opinion, and coming up with a response to your questions will give her some time to digest the idea that you are even considering having sex.

You always want to stick to the facts first, and not overwhelm them with more information at once than they need to digest. Keep an open mind, and don't give up trying. We really want to talk to you too. We are just not always sure how to make our approach.

Make it a Threesome

Sometimes there is power in numbers. Ask a friend whom your parent is aware of to come to your aid and be an ally for you to avoid a potential battle. See if the three of you could be involved in a conversation that perhaps you feel uncomfortable discussing with your parent alone. Then return the favor for your friend by being there to discuss issues with her parent that she would like to discuss.

CHAPTER FIFTEEN

Just a Few Things I'd Like to Get Off My Chest

1. ORAL SEX IS SEX

From what I understand, nowadays, young people do not think that oral sex is really sex. Some of you think that this concept is just something that older people have a hard time understanding. To your generation, you think that maybe it was considered sex back in the day, in our day, but now, it is not. To you guys, (you young'ens) it just doesn't have the same meaning. It's just a casual thing, and really no big deal.

Whether you call it a Blow job, Head, Doming, Slobbing on Bob or the knob, Oral Sex is sex. Hello?? Is anybody listening? It's even in its name. 'Oral' means of or involving the mouth. Sex is performing an

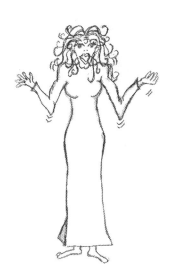

intimate act. The fact is, you are performing a sexual act with your mouth. Rather you choose to believe it or not. You are essentially having sex with someone in the hole in your face.

I mean really. Just think about it for a minute. You are inserting into your mouth, an instrument that is used to eliminate waste, (urine, semen, and other bodily fluids) and do you even know where it's been before? Or what might be lurking on it that could make you sick or that you could share with others? What if he's on the "Down Low" (secretly having sex with men) and his penis just came out of some guy's behind?

Would you go around picking up men's fingers and sucking on them? I don't think so! I mean, really. Why does that seem more disgusting than putting his penis in your mouth?

If you happen to be someone who indulges in this practice, for attention, popularity, fun, or whatever, then honey, you really need to find something better to do with your mouth.

Speak out to help right a wrong. Sing a song , or praise the Lord. Use it to cry out for help because it really is a self-esteem issue.

What you are telling guys is "come on over and use me to dump your trash in. I don't care much about myself, and hey, any attention is better than none at all. Right?" Surely you can find better ways to use your mouth. Especially if the guy doesn't even care about you for real.

And don't think that having oral sex will make him like you. He'll only like you while you're doing it, and when he wants you to do it again. He's more than likely just using you for his own selfish pleasure. He'll tell his friends, and then they'll be asking you to suck on theirs too. Is that the image you want people to see of you? Is that really the visual image you want in peoples' heads?

Girl, your mouth is literally too close to your brain for some of that intelligence not to have better influence over it!

You can still be a virgin and give blow jobs sure, but that just makes you a virgin with a Potty-Mouth and a lot less innocence. This is a much more intimate act, and if you decide to indulge, then surely this should be the thing you hold out for to do with your husband. Giving head should not be used as an alternative reward for not having intercourse. If he loves you, really loves you, he will wait for it all.

Bottom line, Oral Sex is Sex. I know you are familiar with this saying:

"You are what you Eat."

Don't be a (you know what). And don't eat trash.

2. WHAT EVER HAPPENED TO DATING?

It seems that romance is something only found in romance novels these days. Or in the movies, if you can find one. That's unfortunate. If you girls have no desire to be romanced and swept off your feet to the point of floating, then you have no idea what you are missing! Nowadays, people just hang out or hook up, or have 'friends with benefits'. There doesn't seem to be much interest in serious dating or committed relationships.

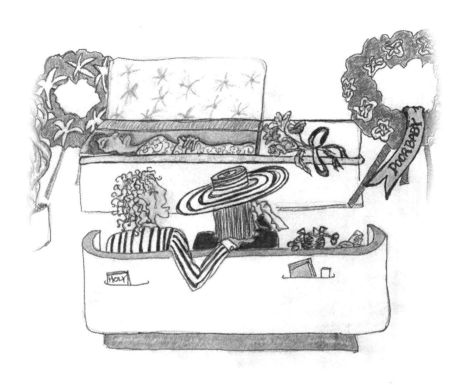

"Well... she always said
he was to die for."

Most would agree that Middle School and even High School is too soon to be involved in a serious relationship; however, to begin to have exclusive relationships later in high school gives you a small taste of what being in a committed, one-on-one relationship is like.

It could be a sneak peak at what marriage would be like. It would be totally wrong, of course, because dating, especially in it's early stages, barely resembles marriage at all. But at least you could have a taste of what it feels like to commit yourself to one person who shares a reasonably close mutual feeling for you.

The thing that concerns my generation is that at the rate some of you younger people are going, especially with these casual connections, and unprotected sex, you may not be around to experience what the flip-side to that would be like.

Everything is just so casual. Not that there's anything wrong with casual dating, it's the casual sexual encounters that worries your parents. Don't you want more than that? You certainly deserve more than that.

If hooking up with someone meant that you could become seriously ill or pregnant, especially if you are not practicing safe sex, wouldn't you want more of a commitment? If not, Why? Wouldn't you want someone that would care enough about you to take care of you when you were sick, to still love you through your multiple personalities of pregnancy, or show up at your funeral with flowers?

Back in the day if a guy was F-I-I-I-N-E... You know the kind where you hyperventilate over him and make those funny quick screams about? Yeah, that type. We used to say, "Oh my God, He's to Die for!" These days, that statement couldn't be any closer to the truth. Women are literally dying as a result of having unprotected sex with a guy just because he was a "cutie pie", or sometimes, just because.

Hopefully you don't think so little of yourself that it doesn't even concern you. Because it should. You deserve the opportunity to have the kind of life you want and you shouldn't allow anything or anyone from seeing that you have it. Especially horniness.

Call me crazy, but if sleeping with somebody could potentially cause my death, I sure as heck would want to know that he'll at least cry for me at my funeral.

Again, our sexual needs and desires can be controlled. It may be hard sometimes (no pun intended) but they really can be. They just don't want you to know it, or even believe it. They are stronger at times and it may seem like we just can't control them, no matter how hard we try.

Try harder. The more you give in to those desires, the more powerful they become. Stop feeding them, and they'll die.

3. FIGHTING MAD

One thing that has always bothered me is why women fight. Especially over stupid stuff, like "You think you're cute" or "that's my man." If someone spreads a rumor around about you, be the bigger person. Go up to that person, ask them, deal with it, and move on. What is fighting over it going to prove? If you get off on bullying and hurting other people, then do it for a career and at least get paid for it. Or win a medal, a trophy or something!

Maybe it's just the crowd and the attention you like. Professional Boxing has a paying crowd. Unless you plan on making it a career, who really cares if you win or not. All you're doing is making yourself look like a jealous, stupid, bully who is so petty you would fight over whether someone thought they were cute or not.

And over a man? Please. Yeah, there aren't that many good ones out there, but the good ones wouldn't involve you in a love triangle either. Fighting over a man does two things. It demeans you further by making someone who has hurt you deeply see that you love being treated so bad so much, you would fight to keep it coming.

Secondly, it forever changes the way the man looks at you.

You don't hear guys telling their boys "These two young ladies were exchanging blows over me." Instead you hear "Man, those B...s were throwin' down!" You don't want to be the B word... You are royalty remember?

I'm just sayin'. I guess I needed to vent a little to work out some of my unresolved issues. I just hate to see women hurting other women. We do that enough already with words.

"Reckless words pierce like a sword,
but the tongue of the Wise brings healing."
– Proverbs 12:18

What bullies really need is a hug. If you want to disarm one, shut one up, or take the confrontation to a place where the bully will have no where to go but to look stupid, just give them a compliment. Say something really nice about them. And mean it. Ask them who hurt them so badly that they would now act the same way towards someone else. Or offer them a hug if you're brave enough.

A lot of bullies that torment and fight people are having the same things done to them by someone else in their lives and they are taking it out on you instead of the people hurting them. If you start to look at your bully as a victim in desperate need of love, maybe it will be easier to be the bigger person and walk away. Or make a new friendship.

4. DRESSED TO KILL

There was a time when that saying "dressed to kill" used to be a good thing. You could be dressed so sharp and look so good someone could fall over and die just out of excitement. You could look so good, a heart could stop beating.

Now, the only killing that's being done is that of the imagination of the men who no longer need to have one. Everything they fanaticize about or would want to, is just as plain and exposed as the nose on your face.

Nothing is left to the imagination. Men are visual and also like to use their imagination to get aroused. They like to try to visualize what's underneath your clothes, and what's underneath your underwear. By you showing them everything already, that takes all the fun away and also could give the message that you must want them to see that and so much more.

Strip clubs are popular because there is a teasing in the slow reveal. The peeling away of layers. There is excited anticipation in the mystery of what lies underneath, and then underneath that. A woman who initially walks on stage as naked as the day she was born will be noticed, applauded and whistled at, for sure.

But the woman who comes out dressed (or at least more dressed than the others) will excite and arouse the crowd more and get their juices flowing. She will be more memorable because men love a mystery. They will remember the naked lady, but the one who came out dressed like a policewoman and then stripped down to nothing... will be remembered with more enthusiasm.

Men want to imagine and fanaticize about what you have. They don't need to have it already exposed and put out there for the world to see. And they want to believe they are the only ones special enough to see it.

The way some young ladies dress these days is really outrageous. It's like wrapping a Christmas present in clear plastic wrap, and then putting it under the tree. What's the point? Why would you want to un-wrap something that you can already see ? It takes all the fun out of it.

What's worse is that it's false advertising! The clothes are saying, "Come get me! Here I am! There's one more thing I have to show you. I'm easy, I'm yours, I'm everybody's!" When the truth of the matter is that they want to say, "Please just look at me, I hate being invisible." Or, "I'm okay with looking exactly like everybody else."

Part of the problem is that the availability of clothes that are stylish, fashionable and not-too-revealing, but not what your grandmother would make you wear to church, isn't there.

It seems even the clothing manufacturers have jumped on the "Let's keep women and girls looking like sexual objects," bandwagon, but here's an idea to fix it.

Some of you out there long to be a famous fashion designer. Dream of it in fact. Why not be the one who creates fashion and style for the new woman who has realized her status as a child of the Most High God? Who isn't about showing everything all at once and appreciates being mysterious.

Imagine the impact you would make on the fashion scene, the amount of money that could be made, and most importantly, the impact you would have on empowering other women! The market is wide open. It could be the opportunity of a lifetime. Not to mention a great thing for womankind!

One last point about the whole dressing thing. Everything is not for every body. Some things were made for only super thin people. Some pants were not made to completely cover all of our behinds. We don't need to let everyone (including people in the grocery store or strangers we meet on the street) see what kind of panties we have on, or don't have on.

If you look in the mirror, (and by all means please do look before you leave the house) and you see what looks like a muffin standing in front of you (tight and neatly gathered at the bottom, and then spilling out and over the top) please, reconsider. That spillage, that part of you that wants to stick out and beyond and then bounce and fall over the top of your pants... please keep all of that to yourself.

Talk about Dressed to Kill! That is certainly one thing you could surely do to kill a guy's enthusiasm or excitement, even if he just saw you walking down the street. That is one of the most unattractive looks you could display, and one certainly that will scare anyone off whether you intend to or not.

Sometimes too much of something (like your stomach flapping over tight jeans) is just way too much of a really bad thing. Try a longer top. Or looser jeans. It would greatly be appreciated by men, women, and children alike. Stop scaring people and grossing them out.

There. I've said it.

CHAPTER SIXTEEN

In The Mean Time...

Okay. So you're buying it so far. You know that you are valuable, worthy, blah, blah, blah. You may even give letting the guy pursue you a chance. You may even find your voice and use it. So what should you be doing in the mean time, during that in-between time while you're making sure that you are ready to take that next step? Here are just a few suggestions to consider.

Maybe a hidden talent will be uncovered. Perhaps a rising star will emerge. Who knows, doing any one of the following instead of giving your body away may even fill that void in you that we are trying to fill with so many other useless things.

Make a commitment to yourself to give at least two of them a try. Watch the magic as you realize how wonderful and phenomenal you truly are! Go crazy, try them all! Have a wonderful journey on the road to discovering yourself, and having the life you really want.

1. GIRL, YOU MUST BE DREAMING.

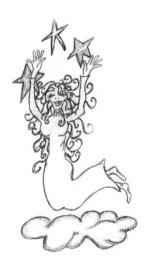

Everything begins with a dream. In fact, every single one of us began as a dream of God. Everything you see, every invention or technique began as a dream in someone's mind as they pondered and visualized the possibilities of what could be.

Even before He created the Earth, surely God had in His mind how this whole earth thing would work, and He saw it and made it exactly as He'd envisioned. (Although, personally, I believe He'd hoped more people would believe in Him and follow Him, but knowing God, that's just all part of the plan.)

Every one of us has the ability to dream. Even people who came out of comas reported to have dream memories. A lot of us choose not to. If you believe, as you should, that having a dream and pursuing it is the reason why we're here, then why not start the process now?

You become what you dream of being. You may not be able to predict your future, but you can certainly create it by dreaming it into being. See yourself in the possibilities of what you want for your life. Then you get all the bonuses that come along with your dream that you never even imagined.

If you really listen to people who had dreams of "Making it Big" someday, their stories go pretty much the same. As far back as they could remember, they had dreamed of being or doing what they are now blessed to do. They practiced, studied, and pursued that dream. At times, it seemed like nothing else mattered. They saw themselves living in the dream. They knew what it looked like, and what it felt like. They believed it was possible!

When asked, what do people always say when their dreams came true? "It's even better than I imagined!" Wow. Imagine that! Dream Big and know that God has an even bigger dream for you.

DON'T KNOW HOW TO BEGIN?
Here's a quick exercise to help get you started.

1. The first step is discover your passion. Think about and then list five things that you love. The things that bring you the most joy. What would you spend most of your time doing if you could? What do you do that makes you feel alive?

(Note: If you can't come up with all five right away, think about things people have told you that you are really good at.)

2. Once you have identified your passions, and know what it is you love, next to each of the five items listed, write down something that you could do with it that could be the ultimate!

For example, if you said baby-sitting brought you joy, then owning the first ever 24-hour daycare center Extravaganza that was so popular there would be a waiting list to get in, and you were about to franchise, so they would be all over the country, and you will never have to work again... that would be the ultimate.

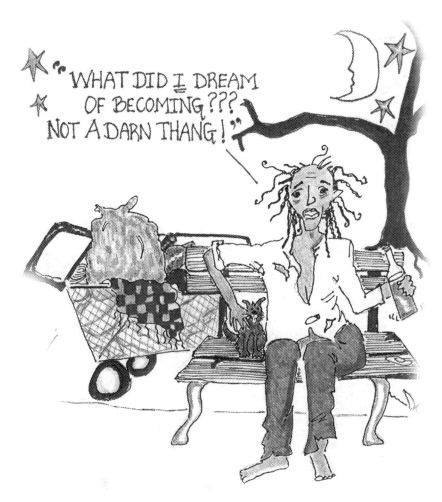

Your Dreams Create Your Reality.

Do that for each item and take what you can do to the limits of your imagination. Beyond what appears to be possible. Then ask yourself what you can do today, to move you closer to that dream.

3. Visualize it. See yourself doing what you love and the joy it brings to others. Walk in it. Cut out pictures in magazines of homes you'd like to live in and imagine how it feels to live there. Do you have an ocean view? How do you feel listening to the sound of the ocean and having your face kissed by the mist of the sea?

Write about what a day in your perfect life would be like. How would it begin, who would be there, and how do you feel?

4. BELIEVE it can happen, and it will.

HELPFUL HINT: *Include in your visions how fulfilling your Dream will be a blessing to others. In other words, how can having your dream come true benefit others? Think of the Big Picture and how many lives can be touched in the process. How many people would now have jobs they love too?*

Dreaming is about putting yourself in your ultimate fantasy and then believing above all else that it can happen. If there is one thing you can certainly do to help create the life you want, the first thing you have to do is see it. Therefore, I say again to you… "Girl, you must be Dreaming!"

II. DO WHAT YOU LOVE

Instead of spending time talking about somebody on the phone, chatting with "stranger-friends" on-line, or zoning out in front of the television, spend some time doing the things you really love to do. If you don't know what that is, then you really need to take some time to find out.

Do you love to sing? Dance? Draw? Whatever it is, spend a lot more time doing it. Whether it's taking care of children, puppies or other people, figure out what it is you love to do, and spend more time doing it.

No excuses. If it's acting you want to pursue, practice going into different characters, or reliving scenes from a movie to your family, friends, or just in front of the mirror. Audition for a role in your school play.

Tell the pastor at your church that you'd like to perform a scene from the Bible. Do what ever it takes to get to the point when you can do it. And then, do it.

III. TAKE AN ADVENTURE

It is such a great big world out there, so big that you have no idea really. What's sad to me is that we don't see a lot of women wanting to explore the world around them, or even what's right around the corner. The days of trailblazing, pioneering women seem to be a thing of the past. But it's not because everything has already been discovered. Here are a few things you could explore:

Yourself

Quite a fascinating creature, yet very misunderstood at times. Do what you can to better understand what makes you who you are, and uniquely you. This discovery can be made in a number of different ways like keeping a journal, meditating, and doing a lot of self-reflection.

Take a deep journey into the heart of you and discover, really discover who you truly are. Spend some very quiet time alone, just listening to what is going on inside of your head. God speaks to us in the silence.

Your History

Shake down the family tree. See what other nuts fall out. Ask questions about where you and your people come from. Older relatives love to share their stories. Do yourself a favor and listen. There may be some things about your ancestry that could make you proud, or want to change your name. Uncover the mystery of how you came to be the person you are, what traits were passed down through the generations, and what you're made of.

Your Neighborhood

So many fascinating things are usually found just around the corner. Explore a new street, a new store or a little known treasure. Go to a local museum and increase your brain size by adding more beauty and information to it. Broaden your horizons, step out of your comfort zone. Turn off the television, go outside and meet your neighbors.

Turn on and watch the news. Not just the local stuff. The evening news. See what's going on in the world. Be informed. Don't be content to just go through life with limited knowledge and information. Education is not always a right or a privilege for all people, and should therefore never be taken for granted.

Take control of your own education. How much you learn is up to you. If you don't know what a word means, look it up. If somebody mentions something that you've never heard of before, find out more about it. Expand your knowledge of this wonderful world we live in, and see how much better you will feel as you gain new information. It really is a powerful thing!

Expand your vocabulary. Have you been using the glossary in the back of the book for words that may have stumped you? I knew a girl who read a page from the dictionary each day in order to increase her word power and usage. Impress yourself and others with words you have newly discovered. Play scrabble! There are far too many wonderful words from which we can choose to keep from using the same tired ones over and over again. Especially of the four-letter variety. Discover new words and use them!

IV. COMMIT RANDOM ACTS OF KINDNESS

It's truly amazing how good you feel doing something unexpectedly nice for someone. Even if they are a total stranger. The real beauty of that is that the person on the receiving end usually turns around and returns the favor to someone else.

I believe it's called "Paying it Forward". If you want to feel incredible or just connected to the human race, try it and you will find it could be contagious. These days, there is so much discussion and coverage of random acts of violence, why not counter all that negativity with random acts of kindness?

Clueless about what to do? It could be as simple as holding the door open for someone or picking something up that someone dropped. Taking a shopping cart back for a mother with a small child. Giving a sincere compliment to someone to brighten up their day. Returning something back that was out of place, or turning something in to the lost and found.

It could be striking up a conversation with a senior citizen (most of them are craving for someone to listen to them and share their fascinating stories with). Who knows, you just may learn something in return. Surprise an elderly relative with a phone call where you are just calling to let them know you were thinking of them.

It could be as simple as reading to a child. Or making them feel really special if only for a moment. You could even surprise your mom by cleaning up the house, (or at least your room) without her even asking.

The point here is that it could be anything as long as it's kind and it doesn't have to cost a thing. The fact is, the rewards you get for doing it cannot even be measured. It feels really good to do something good. Trust me. Passing on a little joy and kindness is very contagious. Most importantly, you will be a better person as a result. Striving to do better and be better is one of the things that we should never stop doing. And best of all… the kindness finds it's way back to you! What you put out, always comes back.

Try to do at least five each day. (Yeah, you can do it. It's very simple really. Just practice being nice.) Watch how the blessings come back to you!

We are all so rude to each other these days, sometimes even a "Thank you", "Please" or a "You're Welcome" would be an act of kindness. (Doing five of these shouldn't count as your 5, though.) Practice these things daily so that being polite and having common courtesy becomes second nature. You'll be a better human being as a result. Thank you.

V. READ A BOOK – OR SEVERAL

You would be so surprised how much you could learn, how far you could go, both in imagination and life, if you allowed yourself the pleasure of reading. The written word can be so moving, so beautifully strung together, so powerful. It could bring out emotions in you that you didn't even know you had. It could open a whole new world of who you are and who you'd like to be.

Do yourself a huge favor. Commit to read (and finish) at the very least three books a year. Start a book club among your friends you hang around with and then you can have something really interesting to talk about instead of "What she said about so-and-so." Expand your mind, your world, and your vocabulary.

Ask one of your teachers or a librarian what they would recommend if you are not sure where to start. There are books that are "classics" that everyone should read, and you are doing yourself a disservice if you make it to adulthood without reading at least some of those treasures.

Reading is giving a gift to yourself that will never lose its value. And it can give you information and knowledge. Knowledge is power! The more knowledge you have the more powerful you become. And you were made to be powerful.

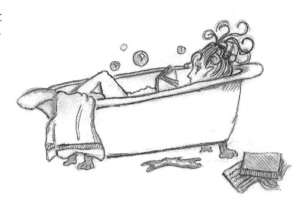

VI. STUDY OTHER GREAT WOMEN

There are literally hundreds of remarkable, incredible women who have done some awesome, inspiring and courageous things, or survived some seemingly impossible obstacles and conditions. Some have made possible the rights that we enjoy today. Study them, learn from them and let them inspire you to greatness. Who knows, maybe we will read about you someday.

Here are just some of the many women you should know and learn more about.

Maya Angelou	Helen Keller
Audrey Hepburn	Ruby Bridges
Sojourner Truth	Martha Cotera
Rosa Parks	Fantasia
Mother Theresa	Sacagawea
Oprah Winfrey	Harriet Tubman
Madame CJ Walker	Hillary Rodham Clinton
Betty Maria Tallchief	Cleopatra
Margaret Mead	Indira Gandhi

VII. CREATE THE MAN OF YOUR DREAMS

Hopefully, I have developed enough creditability with you so far where my mental stability is concerned, because I'm about to share something very private, and I don't want you to think I'm crazy. Actually, I can't believe I'm even sharing this. Only a few people in the whole world know this about me. Maybe it can help someone, I don't know.

As far back as I can remember I've had a vivid imagination. I could dream a dream so real; I could actually see myself in it and feel what I'd be feeling. Like the warmth of the sun on my skin as I lay beside my beautiful pool and the peace and tranquility I'd feel as I listened to the sound of water dancing from a fountain that flowed into the sparkling water of my beautiful pool. I could feel the gentle breeze tingling the tiny hairs on my body as it drifted past. I could truly feel it as I imagined myself in it.

My mother left my father with my sister in her arms and me in her belly. As little girls, the only men in our life were usually uncles and male relatives that we'd see at family gatherings. We knew we were loved, but no one was around on a daily basis giving us what little girls need: Daddies who love and adore them.

When I was three, she married again and life became wonderful as that missing thing that I didn't know was missing filled me and completed me even though I didn't know I was empty. We had glimpses of the Family life I'd dreamed of, or had seen on T.V. I say glimpses because my step-father was a professional basketball player, so he traveled a lot.

At a critical time in my budding life, we became fatherless once again. It was really painful this time because now I knew what I was missing. I needed someone to protect me, love me and laugh at my stupid jokes. It was gone again. And this time I really felt it.

I knew that I had to do something to get that feeling back. To feel the love of a man and know the security that comes with that. So I did the only thing that I could do, and the thing that I do best. I used my imagination and created him. Okay, here comes Crazy.

I imagined the perfect man for me, and he was everything I needed when I needed it. He was my shoulder to cry on, and my friend I could count on. He even taught me the art of kissing, and from what I hear, he was an excellent teacher. Kissing really is an art, and who better to practice on than someone who was always there. And perfect. In every way that a man could be perfect. He had all the necessary body parts, or so I'd imagine, and they were perfect too!

This man was so real to me, I could actually feel his arms around me. We talked about everything. Even the secrets that I'd promised not to tell. We traveled to many places, and he helped me get through the heartaches, hurdles and pains of my teenaged years. And I got to sleep with him every single night.

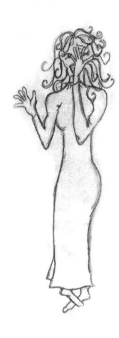

The dream-man I'd created was simply my pillow that magically transformed each night to be the man I needed him to be in that moment. When I needed the comfort of a man and a real one wouldn't do. I knew I wasn't ready for that.

Now you see why I don't tell no body? Right now, in between the laughter, you're probably thinking "I know she did not go there." Well yes, girl, I actually did. He even had a name. Mr. Pillow Man. And he was all mine. And I really loved him because he really loved me.

Even though by now you may think that I am crazy more than just a bit, and this situation may be somewhat amusing, (as it clearly should be when you add the visual) just hold up a minute and let me tell you what happened.

In order to really understand where I'm coming from, you must first know a few things about me. It wasn't that I couldn't get a real man, I didn't have a problem where that was concerned.

Also, I was quite outgoing so I wasn't too shy to let a guy know that I was interested. I just really wasn't. They were just too complicated for me. Caused too many problems. I had problems with people I didn't even know. Coming from other schools and stuff. The guys just never seemed to be worth all the trouble. Besides, I was in training for the day the real one would come along.

Pillow man was my answer to all of the madness. He filled that void, that missing space now aware of it's existence. And like I said, he was perfect. As I got older, so did he. He comforted me and showed patience when my flesh boyfriend wanted more from me than I was ready give him. He held me close and said I was worth the wait. I knew that I wouldn't settle for any less than the beautiful way that I felt.

He was there when I needed to punch someone in the face, and he just took it and let me get it all out. When I was wrong about something, he wouldn't automatically take my side. He would just listen, let me know I was wrong, and tell me he still loved me anyway. Yes, Mr. Pillow Man was the very best of all men put together, and I wouldn't be where I am today without him.

He was fine, strong, loving, tender, generous, kind, and all of the qualities you hope for in a man. He was the closest thing to perfection that I could imagine, because I'd made him that way. He always said what I needed to hear when and how I needed to hear it. And best of all, he absolutely adored me. And loved me like he'd never loved before, and he told me so all the time.

Sometimes I would leave real dates to rush back home to Pillow man (I wasn't sprung or anything like that... trust me, you would have left too) because he was so much better than anything out there. And he knew what I needed.

He was a constant in my life, through horrible relationships, even a horrible marriage. Pillow Man became the standard that I looked for in a man and even my ex-husband couldn't come anywhere close. I knew that I had to hold on to that ideal of all that Pillow Man stood for because I knew that he was the kind of man I deserved. I couldn't let go of the feeling that a love like that was out there for me. For years I had been accustomed to that, and I knew I couldn't settle for anything less.

But I don't have to dream that dream any longer. Pillow Man came alive one day and walked right into my life. The dream I'd held on to for years manifested itself to become reality. A real live walking, breathing, breathtaking dream come true. And guess what ladies? The real one is even better than the one I'd imagined! Imagine that!

You can give yourself everything you need in a variety of different or creative ways. Your body and spirit don't have to be wounded in the process. It doesn't have to be a Pillow Man, I'm just telling you what worked for me. At the very least, think of all of the qualities you want to have in a man… the ones that are important to you. Create him in your mind so you will recognize him when he shows up.

If you do decide to create your dream man through your pillow, just remember that you'll both be a little shy at first and you both might be feeling a little silly. Start off by just talking about what you're looking for and then work on practicing some kissing techniques to become a master at the art of kissing. Believe that the kind of man you dream of is out there, and one day you will find him. Or one even better!

Word to the wise: Be careful and specific about what you wish for... You just might get it.

TEN SIMPLE RULES
[To have a happier Life]

1. Seek first the kingdom of God and His righteousness
2. Keep joy in your heart
3. Love, honor, and respect yourself
4. Always seek peace
5. Strive to do better and be better daily
6. Believe in the possibilities of what you can be
7. Find your passion and live it
8. Always be true to yourself and others
9. Live and love each day as if it were your last
10. Dream always… And then believe they can come true

RISE

If, and when you allow it to, this world can bring you down
Our spirits that were born to soar are somehow on the ground

Hear me now and believe these words,
A lesson to the wise;
You already have everything you need to help your spirit Rise.

The power is within you
And it's calling... Can you hear it?
The voice is of your Father
Always listen. Never fear it.

It's calling you for service. And to help your fellow man.
It's the reason that we came here. To love, then, lend a hand.

At times you feel unable
Too burdened by the pain of trying to stay sane
In a crazy world that's filled with lies
hearing only the deafening sound of your own cries
But like He lifts the sun each morning
He too, can help you Rise.

There is greatness deep within you
With a mission to change lives;
Believe that truth and soon you'll see
that greatness in you Rise.

Rise up and speak up
Cry out if that's what you must do.
Step up and make your mark, A needy world needs you.
Your sisters are crying, too many are dying
As the world looks on through blinded eyes
They are waiting for you... To see them, To feel them
To help them... To rise!

Many challenges await you,
Rise up to meet them, Rise up and greet them
Rise up to your lust and your flesh
To beat and defeat them.

Their purpose is to trick you and fill your head with lies,
And keep you from God's plan for you,
Your destiny... To rise.

We were not made to be ashamed and disgusted
hurt and mistrusted, smacked with eyes busted
Minimized, criticized, then put aside..
How long will we allow men to use and abuse us,
Beat and mistreat us

When, my sisters, will we recognize
And how soon before we realize
That WE are the prize, A Treasure beyond measure
Precious, magnificent and wise
Beautiful, strong and valuable, and worthy enough to Rise

These spirits are heaven bound,
Not meant to drag and scrape the ground,
Silenced or enslaved, or destined to an early grave
By pregnancies, or STD's. Ladies PLEASE
Remember the words of Maya Angelou,
We are all Phenomenal Women, But... y'all don't hear her though.

Destined for greatness, We are daughters of a King!
With promise beyond measure. We can do most anything!
If we dare to dream...
As long as we wake up to the truth that sets us free
And that truth is the same for you as it is for me

We each have the power within us, to do all that we desire
With the spirit of our Father, to guide us and inspire.

Each and every one of us has potential to reach the skies.
Stay strong my sisters! Believe it and face it
Acknowledge and embrace it
Stand up, Stand out, And Rise!

CHAPTER SEVENTEEN

Phenomenal Woman - RISE

The word phenomenal according to the dictionary means extraordinary, exceptional, remarkable, and unusual, among other things. It also says it is relating to or being a phenomenon, that which is known through the senses and immediate experience, rather than through thought or intuition.

In its abbreviated form, we get the word phenom (Fee-nom) - meaning rare and special or of unique significance. Showing extraordinary ability or promise. An object of sense perception as distinguished from an ultimate reality.

As women, we are all extraordinary and remarkable in our own way, and each of us is rare and special and has a unique significance because of our purpose here on earth. There is no one else like you, and no one else was given your "assignment" or purpose to fulfill except you. Finding that purpose is why you're here.

The definition also speaks about being known and felt through the senses, experienced immediately, not just in our minds through our thoughts, but a feeling so real it's better than the reality we could imagine. The ultimate experience—the ultimate reality. That is what being a Phenomenal Woman is all about. And that is what you already are! (You just need to believe it.)

I have been a fan of Maya Angelou since first reading *I Know Why the Caged Bird Sings*, one of three ongoing autobiographies that I'd read while I was in middle school. It changed my life. I had never been so moved by anything I'd ever read before. And I read a lot. Not only was I captivated by the fact that it was an actual life lived, but that it was told in such a smooth, rhythmic way that I remember being proud that Black people could write that way.

It wasn't until I was in college that Ms. Angelou's "Phenomenal Woman" poem came to my attention. I couldn't help but listen with intensity because my Pan African Studies instructor at the time performed the words as she spoke them. The words glided off her tongue and drifted into my soul and I began to feel and believe what I was hearing.

I knew all too well of the struggles and torment Ms. Angelou had faced as a child and young woman, and had always been inspired by how she'd risen from the ashes. To have endured the life she had, and to write such a thing, and believe such a thing was amazing to me.

I remember thinking how incredible it was of her to give this gift of instilling pride to women of all ages and all generations. To encourage us to celebrate womanhood, with heads held high, and apparent pride. And never neglecting our role to help others along the way. It was .... Phenomenal to say the least.

I became mesmerized as these words seeped into my knowing and awakened a belief that I knew was inside of me all the time, it was just often asleep! I really was phenomenal! And it's okay to be proud of that! To celebrate and cherish that.

It became my mantra. My new belief system. I only regretted not hearing it sooner. How different life might have been had I had the opportunity to have those words from that poem ingrained into my personality when I was younger, around your age, while I was struggling through the trials and mysteries of self-discovery and trying desperately to grow up.

Although my self-esteem was pretty healthy, it would have been wonderful to be able to recall those words at times when I wasn't feeling particularly phenomenal about anything, let alone my self.

I encourage every woman to read and embrace that poem for herself. You may have already heard it or portions of it quoted in movies, or on television. Now is the time when you need to begin knowing how great you really are. To really feel it.

Now is the time to experience your uniqueness in grand and positive ways. To show yourself and the world (or at least the world around you) your phenomenal abilities and your bright promise for the future, because you are the future. How you live your life today determines your future and the future of others as well.

Start right now to believe in the magnificence of you and all that you have to offer. Start recognizing it in other women! And then start telling them so.

As women, we should be edifying (lifting up) one another. Instead, we seem to get more pleasure from putting someone else down and then stomping on their feelings, or making them feel worthless. We devalue ourselves and other women. Nobody wins.

When women put other women down, insult or humiliate them , it comes at a great price. Self-esteem is lost. Confidence is lost. The ones doing the hurting loose the ability to feel really good about themselves, because how could you, really? Lost also is the ability to clearly see the other woman for her true potential or purpose in both her life and their own. Everybody loses.

Putting people down is what losers do. And you are not a loser. You are Phenomenal! You lift other women up, and in doing so, lift yourself up in the process!

No wonder men don't always treat us like we're precious and valuable; we don't even treat our own selves with any respect. The really sad part is that we don't even do it with any dignity. We care so little about ourselves that we don't realize how foolish and ignorant we sound trying to bring another sister down. We criticize others because we're so unhappy in our own lives and so miserable with ourselves that we feel we need to deflect attention from ourselves, and try to put others in the spotlight instead.

Put yourself in her shoes or boots. If the way you feel after a "putdown" is not a feeling you'd like to experience, or the shame and rage that goes along with it, then don't be on the giving end. Because what you put out there will come back on you, some way or another. Guaranteed. No exceptions.

Besides, phenomenal women don't act like that. We recognize the qualities that make others unique and special, and celebrate it with them!

If it's hard for you to hold back on being mean-spirited, you need to take a closer look at yourself and find out what the heck you're so angry about! You are just taking out your frustrations on some innocent bystander in order to make yourself feel better. That doesn't make you better, that makes you a bully!

After that, you need to remember (and practice those famous words spoken so very long ago) "If you don't have anything nice to say, then don't say anything at all!"

My daughter experienced ongoing trouble with a group of girls at her school who couldn't stand her because they say she compliments them all the time and that gets on their nerves. How sad is that!!! Do we not want to hear nice things about ourselves, our clothes, our hair, our personality? Have we really gotten to a point where having someone recognize and acknowledge something positive or kind is a reason to want to kick their butts?

There needs to be a change!

Each and every one of us could begin to make small changes starting today. It's a conscious thing. You must make a conscious decision to take control over your mind.

Oh sure, that road won't always be easy. You will be in a constant battle with those little voices in your head. Telling you to do things that you know aren't right. That don't even feel right. You feed them by doing what they say. Giving in to them even though you know it's wrong. Soon they turn into monsters that you can't control. You know the voices I mean. They'll say something like:

"Girl, go on. Ain't nobody lookin'."

"Who cares what your mother says, she's not here right now."

"So what if he doesn't have a condom? Nothing's gonna happen."

When you listen to these voices trying to guide you down a path you know is wrong, starve them and they will die and go away. When you keep giving in, they start getting cocky. They become bigger and bolder, and make you do bigger and bolder things too. Feed only the good voices, and pretty soon they will take over and may be all you hear. Block and replace those negative thoughts and voices with some of these:

"There is always someone who sees everything I do."

"Whether she's here or not, those are her rules, and I will obey them."

"No condom? Right, nothing is going to happen."

If that doesn't work, this one simple statement silences a multitude of negative voices, and is really the only thing you need to say.

"I rebuke you in the name of Jesus."

Good overcomes evil all the time. It has since the beginning.

Take baby steps towards change each day until you learn to walk, then run, and then take flight. All you need to do is to take that first step and start moving! Make choices in your life that show how much you value yourself. If you're not there yet, then do the work to get there. Do whatever it takes to understand and appreciate you for who you are. Be aware of what you say and what you do and how it could effect others. Make choices that show you are paying attention!

Who else is more qualified than you to speak on your own behalf or in your own best interest? What you need to do is to open your mouth and speak out for yourself. Scream if you have to. Or be silent if that will be more effective. You must believe in who you are, as a woman.

Harness all of the energy, strength and spirit that God has given you. It's already in you, and it's running through your veins. It's time to flip the script! Round up all of that that is within you, and make a stand.

Or like Rosa Parks, just stay seated. One tired woman, tired of racism, hatred, injustice and moving out the way of white folks needing a seat on the bus, decided not to move. Her one act of bravery and defiance sparked the Civil Rights Movement, and through that movement emerged a smooth, handsome, poetic talking preacher named Dr. Martin Luther King, Jr., a modern day Moses, demanding our Government to "Let his people go".

Because of her, a man fulfilled his destiny. In his destiny was a dream, and his dream forever changed our world. Because of this one woman, and a personal choice she made that day, the lives of so many others were and continue to be affected.

Surely Ms. Parks had no idea that her one act would give birth to a movement to bring equality for people of color or divide the nation. Surely never even in her wildest dreams would she have imagined that she would be so admired and esteemed both during her life and after her death.

Surely she couldn't have even thought it possible to be the first woman ever to hold the honor of "Lying in State" in our Nation's Capital after her death, an honor usually only held for The President of the United States. She surely couldn't have imagined that she would be remembered forever for the choice she made on that day.

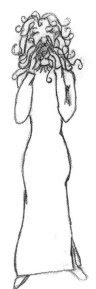

The decisions and choices you make in your life can and will have an impact on the lives of so many others around you. What you do and say and how you act affects your family, friends and neighbors. Think about it. It's like a pebble you throw into a body of water, it has a ripple effect and moves in waves of expanding circles out and extending beyond what you can even see.

You have the ability to touch the lives of so many that you may never know how many lives you are actually affecting.

Your choice may not be as nationally recognized as Rosa Parks, but then again, you never know. Every one of us has the potential for greatness.

And everyone has a voice. Each voice deserves to be heard. Use yours to speak only good things. Only true things. After you speak up for yourselves, find something else you care about, and speak up for that too! Even if just for your dignity and self-respect!

Or speak up to protect the feelings or honor of another person. We need to unify, edify, and celebrate our sisterhood and join together for a common cause. Our value. Our virtue. Our lives.

We need to demand respect and better treatment, and we need to know how to act in order to get it. What we need is a revolution! One that will be televised (You all are much too young to appreciate that statement) —a movement out there for the whole world to see!

Young women all over the world changing laws, and affecting change. Powerful. Valuable. Strutting with pride as we walk with our heads (and panties) up, being the Phenomenal Women we were made to be.

Not long ago a small group of young women boycotted a brand of T-Shirts from a very popular retailer because they felt they were degrading to women. Their act received national attention. I think the store got the message. You could do the same about the degrading way young women are treated.

Sometimes our protests to affect a change or take a stand are more personal, more silent, and are based just on the principle of something. Kind of like our own private platform.

We don't need a crowd or attention from the media.

There are two such silent protests that I have been honoring the majority of my adult life. One is simply for the beauty of our planet. I refuse to litter, or allow anyone in my presence to. I personally think it is so selfish for people to discard their trash any and everywhere and think everyone else needs or wants to see it. I think it's trifling not to find a trash can, and even more so not to even try.

Everyone who knows me knows that if I ever ran out of gas, I would push my car past a Shell gas station to get to the next one because they were the last major company to move away from the Apartheid practices in South Africa.

Sadly, many of you have no idea what I'm talking about, or even what Apartheid means. Lets just say that those of us who wanted Apartheid (the systematic separation and inhumane treatment of Black South Africans from the white South Africans who were actually the minority in terms of numbers) to end, stopped buying Shell Gasoline in protest.

The boycott against Shell ended some twenty years ago, as did the practice of Apartheid, but to this day I have not forgotten their refusal to give equal or fair treatment to my South African brothers and sisters.

While I am sure that they have not missed the little money I would have spent on gas, as a matter of principle, I still refuse to support them or purchase their products. Some things are just harder to get over.

What cause do you feel strongly enough to take a stand for?

Rise up, phenomenal woman and take a stand for something!!!

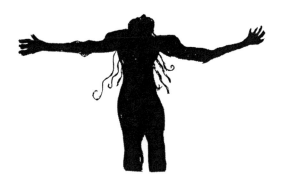

CHAPTER EIGHTEEN

Time For a Revolution . . .

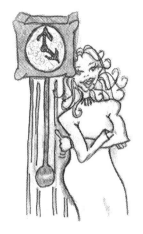

The dictionary describes Revolution in this way: To roll back, to revolve. An alteration or change in some matter or respect. A sudden radical or complete change (in thoughts). Or, an overthrow of one government or ruler and a substitution of another.

We need to start a revolution—a revolt against the current way of thinking about ourselves. To roll things back to a time when women had value and worth. We need to make a sudden, radical change in the way we treat ourselves, and the way we treat each other as well.

We need to revolve—to go around the current way of thinking and get over to the other side! Change the laws in our society to give harsher sentences to those who commit crimes against women, especially young ones. And when you're old enough, vote for those that are sensitive to women's issues and rights and can make changes on a governmental level.

You have a whole world of sisters out there with their own personalities, their own issues, and their own special lessons to teach you. That's the reason they are in your life in the first place. We don't always have to get along, there is usually rivalry among the siblings... but we should still love each other. We should still have each other's backs.

Some young women are lured into gangs because of the desire to be in a group that provides the elements that may be lacking in their own families: like protection, loyalty, and love. Not to mention a feeling of belonging somewhere and having a role to play while you're there. These girls are their family by the ties that bind them, and the intensity of their belief. They are no different than any one of us. We are all just looking to be connected.

Our Revolution can't be seen as a gang though. That word comes with too many negative stereotypes, and negative images. We don't want to scare anybody. We just want them to know we're serious!

What we need, however, is that same level of intensity and loyalty to the cause. The same belief that anything is possible as long as you believe it can be. And we need to believe we are valuable, worthy, and phenomenal, and that soon we will be treated that way!

We could protest and hold up picket signs, and even have a Million Young Phenomenal Women march on Washington. Though effective and powerful at times, these ideas don't offer any long-range solutions or changes that could help us flip this script.

The beauty and magic of this revolution is simply this: You already have everything you need to make that change. You can affect the change. This revolution begins in your own mind. In your own way of thinking. You can make a choice to make wiser choices. Kinder choices.

And that's how we can start a revolution! A movement that will change the values of our lives, and that of our children's and our children's children. We can be Phenomenal women raising Phenomenal women!

Imagine if you would, a time in your future where you are sharing stories with your grandchildren of the Revolution that we started. We are continuing the tradition of passing down wisdom and knowledge to future generations, as is customary to do. As you recall the days and weeks that led to the birth of the Revolution, with great pride you tell them the major role you played. You tell them how the Revolution, the revolt against the then-current backwards ways of thinking, began with one Phenomenal Woman. And that woman was you.

You tell them of the horrors that existed that inspired the revolution in the first place - and of the conditions that demanded it. You describe the incurable diseases that killed us before we'd even really lived. Or of the curable ones that we brought back and shared with as many unsuspecting people as we could.

You tell them how so many young people's lives were gone—quickly snatched away long before their time for reasons that made no sense.

You tell them of the horrible way in which women were treated, used, and then thrown away. And how horribly they treated one another, ignoring the sisterhood to which we should have been united. Instead, women were putting each other down.

You could tell them how the world was filled with angry people who never felt wanted, and how babies were having babies and then more babies. How it was a world full of angry people mad about the decisions that were made by their parents. And the ones they'd made all by themselves.

You tell them how the world was full of lack and longing, and then of violence as a result. How some just took whatever they wanted because their anger made them feel entitled to do so. A world taken over by the 'have not's' destroying all in their path, as if to get back at society for the frustration of existing, and not really living.

You could tell them how awful it felt being invisible and needing to be validated. And appreciated. And loved. How truly awful it felt just wanting to be loved and not finding it anywhere, not even within our own selves.

As your grandchildren begin to squirm and wiggle in discomfort hearing of this distant, frightening world that no longer exists, they move in closer to you. Both fearful and amazed, their eyes look upon you with wonder and excitement and an innocent curiosity to hear how the story ends.

You can tell them that there was no choice. Clearly a revolution was in order. Personally, you had no choice. You believed if you were not a part of the solution, then you were a part of the problem. And your mother did not raise you to be a Problem Child.

Imagine smiling proudly as you reflect on those days, and knowing that this new world, in which women are valued, respected, appreciated and adored, came about because of you.

The ability to look into the faces of your grandchildren, knowing your actions and participation in the revolution provided a future for them is overwhelming. Your eyes begin to fill with tears. You can clearly see that you made the right choices in your life, and they are here because of it.

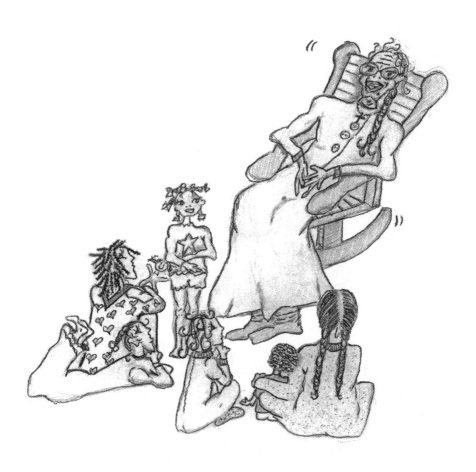

With looks of great pride and enthusiasm on their sweet little faces, they look into your eyes and ask you the question whose answer you have been waiting their lifetime to share with them. The answer that you have already shared with their mothers, and every other woman you have met on your journey into and throughout womanhood.

Their question, simply put was this: What did you do? What role did you play in this revolution that changed the way women are valued and treated in the world today?

You tell them there were only two things that you had to do. Your role was simple and small, but had a huge impact.

The first thing you had to do was just to Believe. Believe in something, and in everything. Believe you are valuable and loveable. Believe you are special. Believe you are a Blessing. Believe you deserve to be treated better, and that some day you will be.

Believe that one person really can make a difference, and believe that one person was you. Believe in the power of womanhood and all that it stands for. Believe that you are destined for greatness. And Believe that dreams come true.

The second and most important role in the movement towards change was your realization of the power found in five little words.

IT ALL BEGINS WITH ME

Change, attitude, a hope for a better life, it all begins with you. The consequences of the choices and decisions that you make, also begin there too. You control where you go with your life, and what becomes of it. What and who you are right now, (happy, sad, angry, used, or delighted) and even what you will become...Starts with you.

You have the power to change any situation just by deciding to change it. Your thoughts create your reality—The greater your thoughts, the greater your reality becomes. Like I said before, you may not be able to predict the future, but you can certainly create it. It begins with your thoughts. Think wonderful thoughts, dream grand dreams and live the phenomenal life you were born to live.

After all, each of us is a child of God, and He surely wouldn't have made us without a very good reason. He never makes mistakes. And you, my intelligent, wise, delightful, talented, beautiful, revolutionary and remarkable young woman... **You** are one of His greatest treasures. All you need to do is to believe that you are! You know… Recognize!!!

Be proud.

Be strong.

Be Bold.

Be beautiful.

Be true.

Be the best!

Be phenomenal.

Believe!

And let the Revolution Begin!!!

Just the FAQ's man
(Frequently Asked Questions)

Can I get pregnant the very first time I have sex?

Yes.

Can you have sex and not get pregnant?

Yes. You can try to prevent pregnancy with the consistent use of condoms and other forms of contraception, but none of them are 100% effective. There is always a chance you can become pregnant even with contraceptives. The only way to guarantee you will not get pregnant is to practice abstinence

What if he "pulls out" before coming (reaching his climax), can I still get pregnant?

Yes. The presence of semen can be found even before the man ejaculates (comes).

Is it painful?

It can be. Even if it's not your first time, it can be uncomfortable or even painful at times. The first time may even produce some bleeding as the hymen (thin layer of skin in the vagina) is broken and you are no longer a virgin. It shouldn't always be painful, and you should consult a doctor if you continue to experience painful intercourse.

It could also be painful if you are not lubricated (wet) enough. This could create a burning sensation on the inside of your vagina and could make urinating painful.

What does it feel like?

Different people feel different things at different times. It's not always as it is cracked up to be, and most young ladies feel a sense of disappointment afterwards, or regret. Especially after their first time. Some feel violated and used, and others feel hollow or ashamed.

The act its self is kind of hard to explain. Two bodies coming together as close as they possibly can, one poking and probing, the other receiving an object into their body cavity. There is thrusting, touching, fondling, kissing and caressing (if you're lucky) and lots of strange and funny sounds being made.

It can be a pleasurable experience, (especially if you have a partner that knows what he's doing, and you are comfortable with him and your own sexuality), but there can also be feelings of pressure, pain or just being uncomfortable. You could feel invaded.

It is an experience you should certainly put off until you are married and ready for all that goes along with it. Let's just say that it is not always as great as everyone makes it out to be. Sex was designed to be enjoyed, but within the confines of two married people. Only then can you really sex at its fullest. It's soooooo much better when you have a sacred love for someone and they feel the same way back!

How will I know if I'm pregnant?

There are signs, some of them old wives tales, some of them are true, but there are several symptoms that could indicate you could be pregnant. You may have any one of these, all of these, or none of them. They are as follows:

A missed period, swollen or tenderness in your breasts, feelings of nausea, (especially to certain smells) or general "flu-like" symptoms. I have also heard that women begin to have this noticeable "glow" that others can see (especially older folks) and you could begin "craving" certain foods.

They have pregnancy tests easily available that could let you know for sure, but you should always seek confirmation and the advice of a professional or another adult. If you become pregnant, find someone trustworthy to confide in. There can be absolutely nothing more frightening than finding out that you are carrying a life that was unplanned, and the consequences of all of your options.

The best way to avoid being in this situation is, of course, to choose to abstain from sexual activity until you are married. Providing financially (on your own and not relying on your parents or the state) for a child is a HUGE undertaking. Know that it requires a minimum commitment of 18 years. So, the next time you get hot and bothered, you really need to ask yourself "Is having unprotected sex with this guy worth at least

18 years of my life?" Statistics show the odds of him being with you to help in all aspects of parenthood are pretty much non-existent. Think about it.

When is it okay not to wear a condom?

A condom should always be used during intercourse (or other sexual acts). It is never okay to have unprotected sex unless both of you are virgins (although you could be told that, and what if it isn't true?) and you are married and planning to have a child. Otherwise, ALWAYS "Wrap it up."

How can I tell if a guy has a STD (Sexually Transmitted Disease)?

Common signs and symptoms of some are the appearance of a sore on the genitals (penis) or genital area, a discharge, or burning or itching in that area. In many cases, however, they don't show any signs or symptoms. This is especially true for women.

Chances are, before engaging in a sexual act, you are not going to examine the guy for sores or ask him if it burns when he pees. Therefore **all** people participating in sexual activity should be tested.

According to the U.S. Center for Disease Control and Prevention {CDC} there are approximately 19 million STD infections in the U.S. each year. Those that are the most infected are women, young people and minorities.

The risk can be reduced greatly by using a latex condom. Female condoms are available also, but they offer less protection.

What if I get an STD and don't know that I have it?

If you continue to be sexually active, you will pass it on to the next guy, and he will effect others, who will infect others, and so on. If you have been active, get tested. Early detection is important. Untreated STDs can cause serious complications including liver failure, certain cancers, infertility (the inability to become pregnant), problems with your brains' ability to function, and even death.

If you become pregnant and have a STD, it can cause serious damage to your baby too, including blindness, deafness, mental retardation and in some cases, even death. It's better to be safe than really sorry. Or dead. Just because someone tells you he's 'clean' doesn't make it true. (Remember the chapter on He Says-You Say? If he says he's clean, you say "prove it".)

What are the chances of getting an STD?

That really depends on you. Every time you engage in sexual activity and have unprotected sex, there is a very good chance you will get one. (The rates are higher for your age group.) If you have multiple partners or a partner who has had multiple partners, your chances are even greater.

If you do not engage in sexual activity, there is no chance you can contract a STD.

How are STDs treated?

There are more than 15 types of STDs in the U.S. They have different causes and are treated differently.

STD's caused by bacteria are often treated with antibiotics (prescription is required). STD's caused by parasites (yes, parasites) are often treated with over-the-counter medicines. STD's caused by viruses cannot be cured. They remain in the body and symptoms periodically re-appear. Treatment in this case is focused on relieving symptoms and reducing the frequency of another outbreak.

You will also have to give the names of your sexual partners so that they can be contacted and treated to prevent the spreading of the disease. Embarrassing, but necessary. If you get treated and your partner does not, you can be infected again.

People in your age group don't think any of this could or will ever happen to them. That's what everyone thinks until it actually does. All of them would tell you that in the end, it really wasn't worth it.

This should make you wonder if having sex, especially unprotected, is really worth the risk. It would be awful to get something from a guy that stays with you longer than he does.

What is the big deal about waiting?

It could be a matter of life and death. Literally. There are so many other things you could be doing with your life, for yourself or for others. Waiting makes you special and unique (especially these days). It also gives you more time to develop the maturity and tools necessary to handle all of the emotions and changes you will go through when you become sexually active. Besides, it's the right thing to do.

Most people do it for all of the wrong reasons anyway..."Everybody I know is doing it," "I just want to know what it feels like," "I'm ready to be a woman," or "I love him."… Just to name a few.

Prove to yourself that you are strong enough to resist those urges, discover more about your self, and work on having a future. Discover your value and believe that you deserve to have a better life than the life being sexually active can offer you. You will have lots of time to experience all that you feel you are missing, and it will be much better if you wait. You don't want to be "used up" by the time the man of your dreams comes into your life. Save yourself for someone really worthy of you and willing to make a commitment.

Besides, what's the big deal about not waiting?

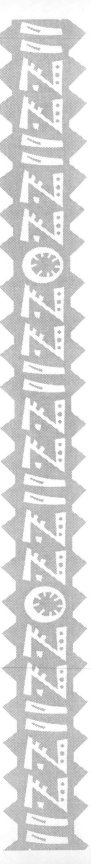

GLOSSARY

Admiration [ad mir ay shun]: wonder mixed with delight. Hold in high esteem.

Adoration [ad a ray shun]: to worship and look upon with intense love.

Conscious [kon'shus]: knowing in one's own mind, awareness.

Contagious [kon tay jus]: sharing of a disease by contact.

Contrary [kon tra ri]: opposite, inconsistent.

Demeaning/demeans [de'mean]: to lower oneself.

Depreciated [dee pree she ate]: To bring down the price or value of.

Desensitized [de sense a tized]: Over-exposure to certain things that make you unable to feel it or be shocked or moved by it as one normally would.

Edify [ed if eye] to build up in a moral sense, speak of with high regard.

Ego [ee go]: An exaggerated love of self, bragging about their own achievements.

Elevate [el li vate]: To lift up.

Elusive [e loos if]: hard to catch or capture, to avoid grasp of pursuit.

Empowering [im pow er ing]: To give official authority to—to authorize.

Endangered [in dane jurd]: To bring into danger or expose to loss or injury.

Entitled [in tite eld]: to give a claim to.

Envisioned [in viz und]: to see clearly in ones mind. To have a mental image of in advance of realization.

Exploited [x ploy ted]: to make use of, not usually in a positive way. To take advantage of for ones own advantage or profit.

Fatal [fay tl]: Causing death. Deadly.

Heir [air]: one entitled to receive another person's possessions or property.

Hoisted [hoyst ed]: to act of raising; to lift upward.

Horrific [whore if ick] Something that causes terror. Frightening or shocking.

Hyperventilation [hipe er vin ti lay shun]: Excessive rate and deepness of breathing.

Impoverished [im pov er ished]: To make poor. Poor means of comfortable life. Wanting. Needy.

Incurable [in cure able]: that which there is no cure for.

Instigate [in sti gate]: to spur on and try to start something.

Integrity [in teg ri ty]: Having honesty that is uncompromised. Firm clinging to a code of morals. Sticking up for your values & what you believe in.

Intimacy [in' ti missy]: a *very* close friendship or personal relationship, marked by affection or love, or where sexual liberty is taken.

Intuition [in too ish un]: A fearful suspicious feeling realized in the mind immediately without reasoning.

Literally [lit ter al ly]: According to the exact meaning.

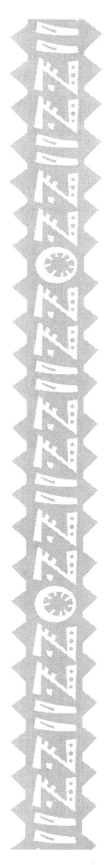

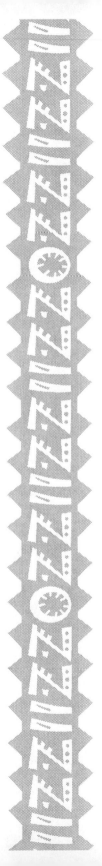

Magnitude [mag ni tude]: greatness, size, importance.

Manipulation [ma nip pu lay shun]: Management with the use of unfair, scheming, or under-handed methods especially for ones own advantage.

Mantra [man'tra]: Speech, hymn, or verbal spell.

Naïve [nah eve]: Marked by simplicity. Showing lack of worldly experience. Innocent. Simple.

Parasite [pair a site]: an animal that lives upon or in another.

Penetrated [pen'a tray ted]: to have entered or pierced, as in another body; to cause to feel.

Perpetrate [per' pe trate]: To do in a bad sense; to be guilty of, to commit.

Perverted [per ver ted]: To turn from truth or proper purpose; corrupted.

Porcelain [pour se lan]: The finest of pottery good.s

Precede [pre' seed]: to go before in time, rank or importance.

Predator [pred a tore] To rob by open violence, To deprive of goods or valuables. violent seizure of goods.

Prey [pray] : A victim. Property taken by violent seizure.

Pulsating [pul say ting]: Beating or throbbing.

Pursuit [per suit]: An act of chasing or going after.

Repels [ree pels]: To drive back. To resist successfully; to cause a dislike of.

Rivalry [Rive al ree]: One who pursues the same object as another. To compete with.

Scenario [sin ar rio]: Plot outline/summary.

Sibling [sib ling]: A brother or a sister.

Statistic [sta tis tick]: The science of subjects and facts calculated numerically.

Trifling [trife ling]: Something of no value or that is taken too lightly.

Ultimate [ul ti mit]: the farthest, extreme

Virgin [ver jin]: a woman who has no fleshy, sensual knowledge of man. Pure, not soiled or polluted.

Virtue [ver chew]: Moral goodness and morality, integrity, honesty.

Vulnerable [vul' ner a bl]: One that could be wounded; open to receive injury.

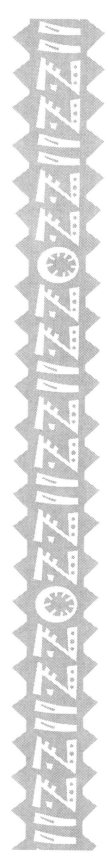

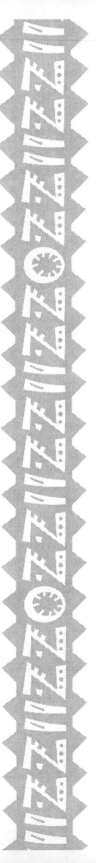

ACKNOWLEDGEMENTS

To my heavenly Father, Thank you for blessing me with the talents you have given me as well as the gift of a heart that cares so deeply about others; and for instilling in me the belief that I could use them both for your Glory.

Natasha Moore & Apostolic Experience Publishing, for not only recognizing the tremendous need for a project such as this, but for also helping to make it one that so closely matched my vision, my eternal gratitude.

Jeaneê & Miles, my most precious gifts, I thank you for your patience, love, sacrifice, and belief in me. I adore you. Your contributions in helping me fulfill this lifelong dream, whether doing graphics for the cover or inspiring me and sharing your friends, I am beyond grateful.

My mother, Barbara Hollier, who showed me the importance of sharing wisdom with your children, and helping to shape me into the woman I am today, my gratitude & love forever. My sister Marla Bradley, for your encouragement and edification, and for your unconditional love, much love and many Smooches! My brother Bill Bridges & his fabulous wife, Lexanne, I am blessed by your love & generosity.

My remarkable cousins, each of whom contributed in grand and phenomenal ways, but specifically Michael Coleman, my constant motivator, and Gary Coleman my constant supporter. Kimberly Merritts, for your input, encouragement, excitement and belief in this project, and your keen editing skills; Markelle Means... Your enthusiasm, interest and assistance to me on this project, giving ideas, encouragement or whatever I needed throughout... For my aunts and uncles, specifically Delores Merritts, and Billy Gaitor, thanks for many years of encouragement, love and having my back! And the rest of my family members who have shown me love, my deepest love and appreciation to you all.

Phoebe Moore, whose simple words of encouragement catapulted me into pursuing writing full-time. Thank you for being the instrument that God used to deliver his message to me.

For phenomenal teachers everywhere who dedicate their lives to plant seeds of hope & inspiration; specifically, Carolyn Cannizzo, my high school creative writing teacher, for recognizing my love and passion for writing and for encouraging me to pursue it. I thank you, and will never forget you.

My life-long sister- friend, Tanya Norrington, whose wisdom, love, friendship and brutal honesty have always been a beacon of light for me, and my forever friend, Marsena Abella, whose belief in me to do this project and all things dreamt of sustained me through even the darkest hours. I am grateful for the connection of our souls as we navigate through life trying to make a difference in it. And my forever love, [Mr. "Pillow-Man"] Thank you for giving me not only the opportunity to fly, but the peace and the comfort of knowing that you'd be there to catch me if I could not. My gratitude and love are eternal.

Lastly, for Maya Angelou, Oprah Winfrey, and all of the great women who have made significant contributions to my life, because of how they live their own; and the spirits of our ancestors, who continue to guide us and inspire. I thank them for speaking through us, sharing wisdom and encouraging us to live a life of purpose. I thank them for their blood that runs through my veins, that leads to my grateful heart. This book is for all of those women, and for those who choose to carry their torch—lighting the way for future generations of women. May we all find value in our selves and in our lives.

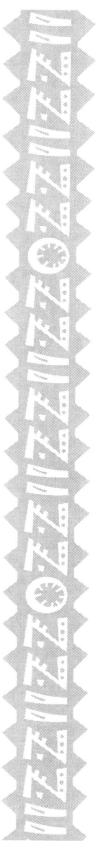

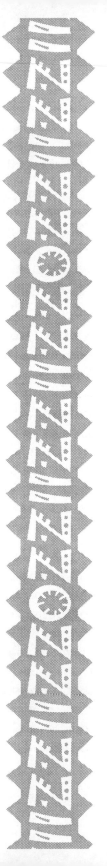

About the Author

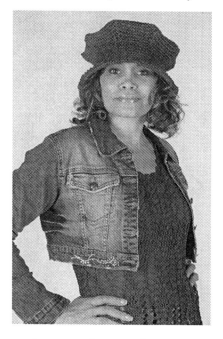

Carla Jeaneê Bradley has literally been in love with words her entire life whether she is reading them, giving voice to them, or simply stringing them along on paper, her love for them is true. Her mutual love of people and her desire to not only study them, but also to enhance their lives, led her to pursue an education in the field of social sciences. She received her B.A. in Sociology in 1984 from California State University, Northridge.

A strong desire to be an integral part of a movement towards positive social change, and a belief that she could do so with her words, led her to pursue a career in writing and motivational speaking. She strives to be at the forefront of the movement to revolutionize the empowerment of young women who truly care about the world in which they live by beginning with themselves.

Carla currently resides in St. Louis, MO with her two teens, Jeaneê and Miles and their wild, crazy, and loveable dog, Bear.

LaVergne, TN USA
24 March 2010

176987LV00003B/23/A